7 WEEKS TO A 10K

7 WEEKS TO A 10K

WEEKS TO A

BRETT STEWART

THE COMPLETE DAY-BY-DAY PROGRAM TO TRAIN FOR YOUR FIRST RACE OR IMPROVE YOUR FASTEST TIME

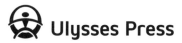 Ulysses Press

This book is dedicated to the memory of Sally Meyerhoff, an amazing spirit and extremely talented athlete who was taken from us far too soon. Smash it for Sally—#SI4S

Text Copyright © 2012 Brett Stewart. Design and concept © 2012 Ulysses Press and its licensors. Photographs copyright © 2012 Rapt Productions except as noted below. All rights reserved. No part of this publication may be reproduced, stored in a retrieval system, or transmitted in any form or by any means without the prior written permission of the publisher, nor be otherwise circulated in any form of binding or cover other than that in which it is published and without a similar condition being imposed on the subsequent purchaser.

Published in the United States by
Ulysses Press
P.O. Box 3440
Berkeley, CA 94703
www.ulyssespress.com

ISBN13: 978-1-61243-188-8
Library of Congress Control Number 2013930887

Printed in Canada by Marquis Book Printing

10 9 8 7 6 5 4 3 2 1

Acquisitions Editor: Keith Riegert
Managing Editor: Claire Chun
Editor: Lily Chou
Proofreader: Lauren Harrison
Index: Sayre Van Young
Design: what!design @ whatweb.com
Interior photographs: © Rapt Productions except page 11 © Kristen Andersen and page 18 © marema/shutterstock.com
Cover photographs: front © Gabriel Gurrola; back © EpicStockMedia/shutterstock.com
Interior photographs: see page 148
Models: Michael Bennett, Brian Burns, Evan Clontz, Lewis Elliot, Brett Stewart, Kristen Stewart

Distributed by Publishers Group West

Please Note: This book has been written and published strictly for informational purposes, and in no way should be used as a substitute for consultation with health care professionals. You should not consider educational material herein to be the practice of medicine or to replace consultation with a physician or other medical practitioner. The author and publisher are providing you with information in this work so that you can have the knowledge and can choose, at your own risk, to act on that knowledge. The author and publisher also urge all readers to be aware of their health status and to consult health care professionals before beginning any health program.

CONTENTS

Foreword

When I was sitting down to write this book, I had my first bout of crippling writer's block—a serious, finger-paralyzing fear that crept over me and prevented me from typing a single word on my trusty little MacBook. My lockup wasn't due to lack of material; I've been obsessing and learning everything possible about running for nearly a decade. If anything, I was overwhelmed by the sheer magnitude of all the research and testing I've done for my own programs and those I've coached my athletes through, all the things I've screwed up and the times I succeeded way beyond my own expectations. Through it all, I've been keeping a mental diary of the places I've gone and every single thing I've seen and done along the way. That's a lot of pressure to condense all those tips, tricks, tidbits, failures, foibles and follies and share them within the number of pages I've been allotted in this book!

In order to clear my head, slice through the glut of material I wanted to present and return my fingers to the keyboard, I decided to employ some sneaker therapy—in other words, go out for a run. With this writer's block really knocking me off-track, I knew I needed to go for a rather long run...so I signed up for one of the premier ultra-distance events in the United States, Across the Years in Glendale, Arizona. After over 50 miles, hundreds of conversations, roughly 100,000 steps and millions of thoughts later, my mind was clear and my writer's block was gone. The answer? I'd write about all the changes that have occurred in my life, how they started with just one step. The day I started to run was the first step to a completely new, healthy, happy and extremely satisfying life.

This book is my humble addition to the world of running, an attempt to give back even a fraction of what running has given me. It would be the ultimate gift if my words encouraged just one person to experience the life-changing effects of running. I sincerely hope this book will help motivate you to take that first step.

—Brett

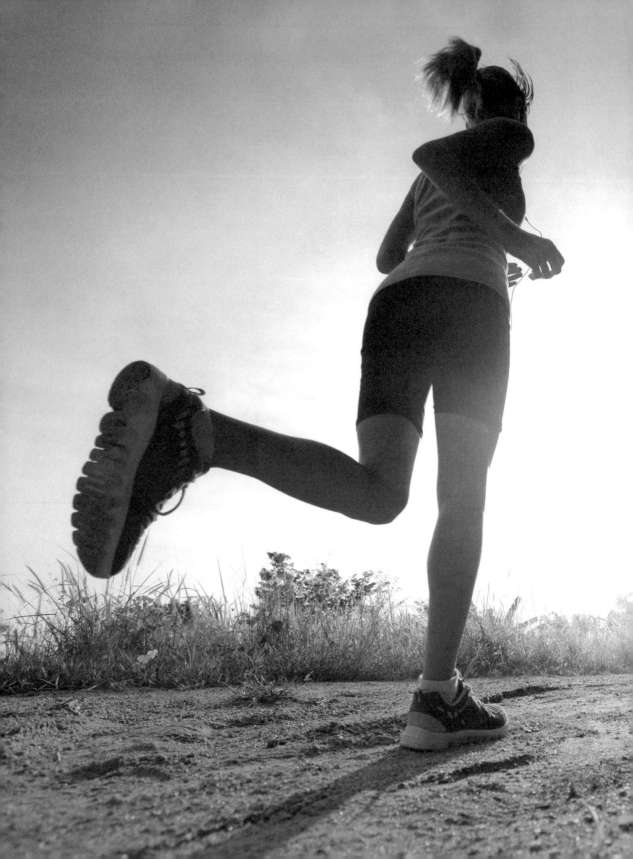

PART 1: OVERVIEW

Introduction

I've been chased by zombies. I've run past rattlesnakes, crossed the raging Colorado River, circled a baseball field repeatedly for over 50 miles, sprinted past world-famous athletes (only to be left in their dust shortly thereafter), and watched a world-record ultramarathon distance get shattered. I've been lucky enough to run alongside Dean "Ultramarathon Man" Karnazes (one of my running heroes and a fantastic guy) in the middle of nowhere in Globe, Arizona, and got lost with him on a trail in Austin, Texas. Heck, I even got to run my first ultramarathon by Karno's side for the first few miles.

Running has taken me to the Outer Banks of North Carolina and all the way to San Diego, both times to run some of the most exciting marathons in my life. I've enjoyed running down the middle of the Las Vegas strip under the Sin City lights past all the billion-dollar hotels, and in the middle of, well, nowhere in Montana. I've seen more places across the United States with running shoes on my feet than I can count, and each experience has been special to me because there's no way I should ever be a runner—I'm just a fat kid from Connecticut.

I'm the second of two boys. My brother was the honor student, all-star baseball player and on the starting basketball team as we were growing up—and I was the one "riding the pine." My athletic prowess (or lack thereof) was only due to my dad taking over as Little League coach and putting me at second base. Willie Randolph, I was not. Aside from being the team mascot cheering from the bench, I was the kid who'd (occasionally) hit a ball to the outfield grass and still get thrown out running to first. Have you heard the phrase "you could time his speed with a sundial" before? Well, that was me.

Pudgy, slow and below average were the terms I'd use to describe my youth, and for the next decade or so it only got worse. By age 29, I was overweight, smoked about two packs of cigarettes a day, and sat on my butt in front of a computer screen for eight hours a day before heading back home and plopping on a couch to stare at the boob tube. My weight had easily eclipsed 200 pounds, and at 5'8" tall, I was the furthest I could possibly be from being an athlete. I had stopped playing sports, wasn't dating and was pretty darn bummed about my life when one of my employees and good friend Chris Goggin challenged me to do a duathlon with him. I tell the story of that adventure in *7 Weeks to a Triathlon*, but prior to showing up for that event, I "prepared" by running my first 5K.

That day in downtown Hartford, Connecticut, a decade ago, my journey to becoming a runner was launched rather inauspiciously. Walk, run, jog, walk, curse, walk some more, trip, tie shoe, walk, run, tie the other #$& shoe and curse a little more...and that was just the first mile. I didn't realize it then, but everything I've come to know and love about running across the years started with just one step. A little piece of me longs to go back to that day and start all over again knowing what I know now, but the reality is that I wouldn't change a single thing. In running, the journey is its own reward, and everything you learn, see and do along the way is a treasure unto itself.

About the Book

Much more than just preparing for a specific 6.2-mile event, *7 Weeks to a 10K* is about all aspects of running. (It would've been difficult to sell a book with a title like *7 Weeks to Learning Everything You Ever Wanted to Know about Running but Were Too Afraid to Ask the Clerk at the Shoe Store*. In Part I, we cover some background on the 10K, explain why seven weeks is an appropriate time to meet your goals and then spend a huge chunk of the book talking about running in general. Case in point, the FAQs only contain one question specific to the 10K distance. As I mentioned earlier, this book is about your journey into being a happier, healthier or faster runner, whether this is your first jaunt into the world of foot races or you're a veteran looking for some tips to improve your fastest time.

The initial section of the book is the proverbial starting line, and Part II is where the show rubber meets the road, trail, track or what have you. In this section, we cover everything you need to know to get out and run—the gear and gizmos you may (or may not) need, mental preparation, goal setting, as well as where, why and especially how to run. This section is all about the pastime, sport and passionate pursuit of running, not, like I said above, specific to any particular distance. Whether your goal is to run a 3K or a 30K (and all the mile equivalents in between), this is all stuff you should know! I even share some other training plans so you have a well-rounded view of the different techniques for starting out and progressing as a runner.

Part III gets specific about training plans. The Prep Program is for first-time runners or those coming back after a break or an injury—the goal is to get off the couch and get active. This program is everything you need to get you into the rhythm of running and a perfect way to practice the basics you've learned in Part

II. The Level 1 Program is geared toward relatively fit individuals who are ready to tackle their first 10K, have finished some shorter-distance events, or have an athletic background. Done a 5K? Start here. In the Level 2 Program we add more intensity in the form of speed work, hill work and advanced cross-training exercises to build a stronger, faster body. Running doesn't take a backseat to all the other exercises— this program is specifically designed to help you drive your running to the next level, be it 10K PRs (personal records) or even longer distances.

In the Appendix you'll find illustrated cross-training exercises, warm-ups and stretches, a training log and a run-down of what to expect on race day. How about a checklist so you don't forget anything on race day? Need one of those? Well, now you've got it.

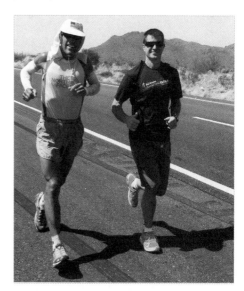

The author running with Dean "Ultramarathon Man" Karnazes somewhere outside of Globe, Arizona, during one of his runs across the U.S.

What Is a 10K?

"Why on earth do we run 5Ks and 10Ks here in the United States? Didn't we reject the metric system?"

—BILL RIBBLE, BRETT'S RUNNING PARTNER

Let me be honest: When I first started running, I didn't know the difference between a 401k and a 10K. Somewhere around mile 2 of my first 5K, the thought of completing a 10K seemed as irrational as climbing Everest in flip-flops. Little did I know I'd be running distances 10K and more in only a matter of months. When you get bitten by the running bug, anything can happen!

Ten thousand meters is a pretty impressive sounding distance, right? Ten kilometers also sounds like a heck of an accomplishment too, while "10K" (pronounced *ten-kay*) is a bit friendlier and quick off the lips. Let's look into the different times this same distance is referred to by these different names.

Ten thousand meters, or "the 10,000," is the moniker for track events around the world. The most prominent of these track-and-field events has been contested every four years for the last century at the Summer Olympics. The longest of standard track events, the 10,000 meters is the equivalent of 25 laps around a 400-meter track. When this distance is referred to as a "10K" and held outdoors as part of track-and-field events, it's considered a long-distance cross-country event.

Most non-collegiate runners are exposed to 10Ks as a mid-distance road race, double the distance of 5Ks and almost 50 percent the distance you'd be running during a half marathon...but that's where road-racing distances switch to miles for measurement and the breakdown gets a bit confusing as mathematical conversions come into play.

Speaking of distance conversions, take a look at the chart below. As you can see, there are a multitude of "common" race distances that take place on roads, trails, sidewalks and paths all over the

Event/Distance	Equivalent
1 meter	.0006 mile
1 mile	1609.34 meters
5K	3.1 miles / 5,000 meters
8K	4.97 miles / 8,000 meters
5 miles	8046.72 meters
10K	6.2 miles / 10,000 meters
15K	9.3 miles / 15,000 meters
20K	12.4 miles / 20,000 meters
Half Marathon	13.1 miles / 20,921.5 meters
25K	15.5 miles / 25,000 meters
30K	18.6 miles / 30,000 meters
35K	21.7 miles / 35,000 meters
40K	24.8 miles / 40,000 meters
Marathon	26.2 miles / 42,164.5 meters
45K	29.9 miles / 45,000 meters
50K	31 miles / 50,000 meters

world. Sometimes even the name of the event itself can be misleading, as is the case with the famous Comrades Marathon in South Africa, which is actually more than double the traditional 26.2-mile/42.2K "marathon" distance. Of course, any race can be any distance long, and that's a lot of the fun about running: "Race you to that mailbox!" The reasoning for standardization and even measured, certified course distances is to develop a baseline for comparison of times, making state, county and even world records viable and even allowing you to compare your time against that of your friends, as well as track your progress from race to race.

Of course, even if the distance is the same, environmental and terrain factors can come into play and skew the results of some races. A hilly course can end up being faster or slower than a flat course depending on the differences in altitude, temperature, wind, surface conditions, timing and length of the hilly sections and so on. Runners may call a fast course a "dog track"; a runner can expect a fast time or even a personal best (PB) on a "PR-friendly" course; a slow course can be called anything from "miserable slog-fest" to a "challenging" course.

Why a 10K?

The 10K is an excellent test of your strength, speed, strategy, planning and endurance. This distance is short enough to be run "fast" (a relative term; we'll cover this later in "Understanding Your Pace" on page 78) yet long enough to

require strength and endurance. In shorter distances like a 5K, experienced runners can usually pin the needle in the red (or somewhere near it) and run close to all-out for the entire distance, while the 10K requires a bit more strategy and planning for when and where runners will push their pace. The longer the distance, the more of a game plan you'll need to race it successfully.

Another reason for the extreme popularity of the 10K is it's often bundled with other races. At a "Five and Dime" (5K and 10K) event, athletes are given the choice to register for either the shorter or longer distance. Those who are new to running or looking to run fast and possibly set a PR will gravitate to the 5K, while runners looking to push themselves over a longer distance and test their endurance and tempo will pick the 10K. It almost goes without saying that there's a teensy bit of bragging rights to doing the longer distance; you're usually treated with a modicum of respect when you're walking to the start line wearing the longer-distance bib. The 10K is also often bundled with half marathons as the shorter distance, and this boosts runners' awareness for this distance by it being the faster, shorter stepping stone to the half marathon and eventually the full marathon.

If you've completed a 5K and are looking for a new challenge, 10Ks are a great step up. For longer-distance runners looking to build their pacing and tempo, break up their boredom and knock through their plateaus, training for and racing the 10K distance is highly recommended.

Why 7 Weeks?

I get this question quite a bit by e-mail and during interviews, so let me be proactive and share the answer with you here. General sports and fitness training for events is a year-round event for a lot of people (me included), and it's extremely necessary to change your routine every so often to avoid plateaus, overtraining, and mental or physical burnout. Even professional athletes take a good chunk of their off-season to engage in different sports or activities and change their workout routines. Guess what? Seven to eight weeks is the optimal window for learning a new routine, adapting to the exercises and the new demands on your body, perfecting the form and reaping the benefits, and then testing yourself (like racing a 10K). You can then transition to a new program or re-load the same program and make some modifications to the intensity, weight or duration.

WEEK 1: Learning the routine. Everyone's a beginner once—don't rush through this part or you'll knock yourself off-track with delayed onset muscle soreness (DOMS) by overdoing it too quickly. Take your time and learn the exercises and proper form by performing them slowly and carefully. This will pay off come week 3 or so, trust me.

WEEKS 1–3: Adapting to the exercises, working through initial soreness and making the training a part of your routine. This actually starts with your first or second workout. Some athletes take 10–14 days, while others need 18–21 to lock it in. During this period, 50 percent of workouts fail because individuals don't rearrange their lives a little bit to make the new program work. Life happens, but you can always come back and pick up here or start over.

WEEKS 3–7: Perfecting the form, seeing the most strength and fitness gains. This is the sweet spot and the reason why you took it slow on week 1 and stuck with it (see "Why does running the first mile suck so much?" in the FAQs on page 20). There will be one or more times during this 28-day period where you feel bulletproof. Remember, you may be a rockstar, but you're not made of Kevlar. Act accordingly.

WEEK 8: Tapering for The Race. If you have a race planned, this is where you'd taper (page 26) and prepare for your event. You'll be running 50% of the distance with lower intensity, just enough to keep loose and active while also allowing for rest and recovery so you're fresh and ready on race day.

If you haven't registered for a race and still want to test yourself without dropping some cash on an entry fee, take a week-long taper and then test yourself in a timed 10K using your watch or race against a friend. It's great to have a benchmark for how far you've come, and there's a good chance you'll revisit the program to ramp up your training now or after a transition week.

If you're using this program for fat loss, body-shaping and sport-specific training, you can transition from the workouts in this book to others (ahem, www.7weekstofitness.com) rather easily. Since this is a running and cross-training program, you should keep running and exercising, just take it down a notch and allow for some rest and recovery. This is similar to the run-specific term "taper"; the exercise version is called a "deload" week. You'll be performing a lighter workload for the next seven days until you start up a new program or jump back into the Level 1 or 2 programs and up your intensity. Follow Week 1 of the program you just completed—this should be roughly 60% less distance, reps and time than the Week 7 you just finished. It'll provide exercise to keep you loose, but a reduced workload to allow you to recover, reset and plan your next goal.

Frequently Asked Questions

New to running? There are hundreds of questions you can ask about the best way to start, what you should do, how you should train, what gear you need, etc. While it may seem like there's so much for you to learn immediately, there's no test for you to worry about. No one's going to stop you at the registration desk for your first race and ask you any difficult questions! Running is actually very easy to get into and hooked on—there's no reason to make it overly difficult or confusing. Throughout this book I'll share information I've learned through about a decade of running and picked up from professional and amateur athletes, coaches and trainers along the way.

Q. How far is a 10K?

A. 6.2 miles. Remember, the first 6 are easy. It's that .2 that'll get you every time.

Q. I hate running. Why did I ever decide to pick up this book?

A. That's a pretty complicated question. There may be something deeply wrong with you in some dark, disturbed corner of your brain. Or you may just want to get fit, challenge yourself, meet some interesting/fun people and develop a new routine of training and conditioning that can help keep you in great shape year-round.

When runners relate the positive aspects of running to non-runners, they usually just focus on the many physical benefits one can obtain from running: improved health, strength, speed, endurance, weight loss, etc. They forget to share how running can deliver some amazing mental dividends, specifically the confidence to build up to your goals with progressive training or a reward only a runner can explain—the elation accompanying the dopamine release that causes a runner's high. We'll cover this a bit in "The Highs & Lows of Endurance Running" on page 72.

Q. Can I walk during training or a race if I need to?

A. Yes, yes. yes. And, furthermore, yes. Walking is absolutely a part of running, especially if you're just beginning. Walking plays a role in training and racing every distance during some point in your career, and there's absolutely no shame in walking, especially if you're sticking to a specific game plan. We'll cover some excellent reasons to perform run/walk intervals and how they can play a critical role in hitting your goals starting on page 77.

Q. Why does running the first mile suck so much?

A. Because it always does. No matter how long you've been a runner and how experienced you may be at any distance or speed, the first mile of training or warm-up is usually one of the worst. Your form is sloppy, usually you have sore muscles from a previous day's training, your back is stiff from the way you may have slept last night or sat in your chair at work with poor posture—whatever the physiological reasons are, there are mental ones too. We'll mention this phrase a couple more times, but here it is: "Embrace the suck." A term used by soldiers in the military for digging deep to complete tasks or finish off their tour of duty and get home, it has been adapted for civilian use. So go ahead and embrace the suck of the first mile or so, you'll be through it soon enough.

Q. Can I use this program while I'm traveling?

A. Absolutely! One of the great things about running is the places it will take you! Personally, I try to sneak a run in each morning on vacation or when traveling for work; I'll ask at a hotel's front desk if there are trails in the area or search online resources. If I have a bunch of time, I'll even try to get lost (but then I always bring my phone just in case!).

Q. What's a tempo run?

A. A tempo run is a pace that's relative to each runner. Basically it's a prolonged run of 15–20 minutes at a speed that's about 30 seconds per mile below your race pace after warming up. Tempo runs are a great way to progressively build speed over greater distances during training. I'll cover more on determining your race pace, perceived exertion and different styles of running in the programs in Part 3.

Q. Will speed sessions make me faster or just tire me out quicker?

A. Both, but that's the whole point! Varying speeds over distances, intervals and even during different timings in your workout will help you to develop the strength, speed and stamina to run faster for longer periods of time. Check out the programs in Part 3 for much more about how we plan on putting this to work.

Q. Why hill work?

A. Varying surfaces are important in training, as very few real-world courses are perfectly flat. Aside from that, hill work sessions will develop leg strength, which in turn will make you more versatile as a runner and more well-rounded to prevent injury. Plus they're a quick, tough workout that will leave you with quite a feeling of accomplishment when you've knocked them out.

Q. Intervals—what are they and why do I care?

A. Intervals are alternating periods of effort and rest, and are key in getting optimal workout results in the least amount of time. I think you'll agree that getting an excellent workout in half the time—with sometimes even more positive results—is a good thing. Of course, intervals require more intensity for those shorter periods of time, but they're well worth it. You'll see plenty of intervals in the programs in Part 3.

Q. Should I take an ice bath after a hard workout?

A. That depends. How much do you enjoy jumping into a tub filled with ice? Some people swear by the reduced recovery time and less inflammation, others say it's just a placebo effect. I say if you can handle it and feel it will help, then go for it. Not sure if you're ready for it? Take an ice-cold shower after your runs and see how long you can stand under the freezing water.

Q. Epsom salts? Isn't that the stuff my grandmother used?

A. While I can't speak for your good ol' Grams, I happen to know of some very distinguished runners who rely on a 15-minute soak in Epsom salts to ease muscle pain and cramps after hard runs.

An Epsom salt bath is a simple, quick, natural and affordable way to facilitate recovery and ease muscle soreness. Purchased at most grocery stores and pharmacies in a container that resembles a cardboard milk carton, Epsom salt is rich in magnesium and sulfate, which are absorbed through the skin very effectively—arguably more effectively than by taking supplements orally. A quick dip in a warm bath with a couple cups of dissolved Epsom salts can aid in flushing toxins from your cells, easing muscle pain and cramps, and eliminating harmful substances built up in your body from the stress of training.

Q. Do I need to overhaul the way I run to get faster/go farther?

A. No. Well, probably not. Some great runners have horrible form, and there's no benefit to trying to change it unless they're seriously working to be in the elite ranks of professional athletes where every single motion is scrutinized by a coach. For Joe or Jane Average? You're probably doing it okay, and a few pointers to help you run a little bit more efficiently will go a long way. I have some tips starting on page 57 to help you improve your form.

Q. I heard that running is horrible for my knees/back/spleen/nostrils/etc.

A. Life is hard on your body, running isn't. Actually, the health benefits of losing weight, adding muscle and increasing your cardiovascular system's efficiency far outweigh the wear and tear on your body from being active. Running is an activity, and all activities increase your potential for injury; that's just the nature of the game. Personally, my knees, ankles and hips have never been stronger since I started running—quite the opposite of running "wearing me down," right?

Q. Will people laugh at me if I walk in a race?

A. Nope, not at all. Then again, anyone who laughs at you isn't even worth your attention anyway. As I mentioned earlier, several different training and racing strategies involve walk and run intervals. I explain more in the progams in Part 3.

Q. My cousin is a great runner. She says I should follow her program. Why would I use this one?

A. Congrats to your cousin, seriously. Some folks hit the genetic lottery and were born with exceptional athletic prowess. The rest of us have to work hard to reach our goals, and there's no easy way to become an accomplished runner. No matter which program you choose to use throughout your running career, it's always a good idea to pick other runners' brains for their training plans, nutrition, tips, advice and tricks. Try the ones you're interested in for yourself and see what works. A lot of the techniques in this book come from a variety of things I've learned from a whole bunch of different runners— some professional and most amateurs. You may never know what advice will work for you until you try it.

Q. LSD? Are you talking about drugs? What the heck?

A. No, in this case, "LSD" means "long, slow distance," or building your base by performing one long run per week. We'll talk about why this is an "old school" idea that may or may not work for you in he programs in Part 3.

Q. Should I stretch before I run?

A. That depends on what you mean by stretching. Yanking at cold muscles and holding them in an awkward position for 20 seconds? No. Not at all. You should never pull on cold muscles unless you're looking for poorer athletic performance or even potentially injuring yourself. You should always warm up first with a brisk walk or slow jog, then some dynamic stretches like the ones we cover on page 135, before you start a hard training session or race. If you're going out for an easy jog, use the first 5–10 miles to warm up, then loosen up a bit with a few of those moves and then continue your run. If you feel tightness in an area while you're running, pause and shake it out or gently stretch it before continuing.

Q. Why am I sore after even a short run? When will it stop?

A. Your soreness depends on your age, conditioning, the intensity of the workout,

terrain, form and countless other factors. The good news: It usually gets better as you adapt to a program. The bad news: As you're progressively pushing yourself to reach new goals, you'll continue to develop soreness after a workout. Post-exercise stretching, recovery and rest will help you alleviate some soreness. The best tip is to get eight hours of restful sleep. We cover some ways to maximize your downtime on page 73.

Q. What on earth is a foam roller?

A. This tube of hard foam is a blessing and a curse: The deep massaging benefits of foam rolling post-workout and after stretching or before bed are many, but it can also be a bit painful. Then again, nothing worth having doesn't come without a little pain, right? Placed on the floor beneath your glutes, hips, hamstrings, calves or quads, your body weight provides the pressure on the foam roller and you roll back and forth to loosen and elongate the muscles, remove knots, and improve blood flow for recovery. Whatever brand you buy should come with comprehensive instructions, and you can also find a wealth of knowledge about foam-rolling techniques online.

Q. Should I lose weight before I start running?

A. Why not let running help you lose weight? The Prep Program (page 88) is an easy way to get into the swing of a routine and will help you walk, jog and run at your own pace to help lose weight and prepare you for Levels 1 and 2 down the road. The best part? It's all relative. You can use the Level 1 Program for as long as you need as you build up your strength and athletic ability and drop weight before progressing.

Q. It's too hot/cold/rainy/hilly where I live. Can I use this program on a treadmill?

A. Sure! Running outside can be a little more exciting than being stuck on a "dreadmill," but I know plenty of runners who log thousands of miles on their treadmills and achieve great results at races. The benefits of getting a run in without worrying about weather-specific clothing can be a big plus when you're strapped for time. One tip: Always change the elevation of your treadmill deck to at least 1 or 1.5 degrees to reduce the flat-footed impact on the belt that can lead to shin splints.

Q. I don't have enough time to run!

A. Yes, you do. That 5 minutes you waited in line at Starbucks, 15 minutes on Facebook before lunchtime and 60 minutes spent spacing out while pretending to be working would be a perfect time to sneak in a couple miles. It's all about finding the spots where you can sneak a run in, and then clean up, change and return to your daily activities. When I was at ESPN, a group of us would run about 3 miles a day at lunchtime and grab a quick shower before heading back to the office and eating a quick lunch. Don't have a

shower? Bring some sport wipes (like baby wipes, without the baby smell) and a little deodorant. It works pretty well!

Q. What should I eat and drink when I run?

A. This depends on the distance of your run. Less than 45 minutes in average temperatures? A little water is all you need to bring along. In extreme heat or runs longer than 45 minutes, a little sports drink to replace electrolytes, salt and sugar is beneficial. For runs over 90 minutes, an energy gel or half of a sports bar will keep your energy up. You'll need to experiment

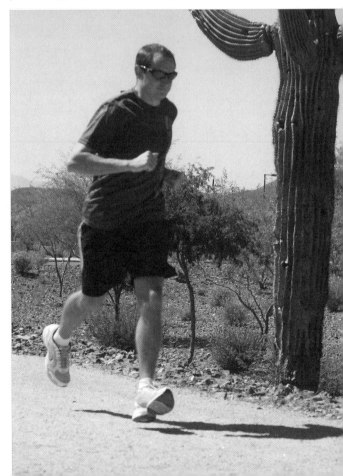

with fluids and solids in training to see how your body reacts so you know how to fuel and what to expect on race day.

Q. What happens if I come in last?

A. You'll get some of the biggest cheers, no question about it. As a race director, I've personally run the last mile or so with the final runners and had a great time watching the crowd erupt when they run down the chute to the line. Spectators are conditioned to cheer for winners, but everyone loves an underdog. Never fear being last—just don't quit or you're robbing yourself of your moment of glory.

Q. Seriously, can I really run a 10K?

A. Why the heck not? I've been lucky enough to race with Army veterans on prosthetic limbs, athletes in wheelchairs and amazingly competitive racers who have lost hundreds of pounds due to the transformative effects of running. I know you can do it—the question is, do you?

Q. Why are runners so crazy?

A. This book isn't nearly long enough to cover this subject. We're all a little nuts. Apparently, something happens right around the time you start calling yourself a runner; you pick up running magazines, spend inordinate amounts of time in the athletic department at stores, shop for the newest running shoes, gizmos and gadgets, and drive your spouse and friends nuts until they either become runners

themselves or turn a deaf ear and blind eye to your obsession. Embrace it—it's a good kind of crazy. Let's face it, there are many habits that are far worse than being an annoying runner. Just don't take yourself too seriously.

Q. Is a treadmill safer for my knees than running outside? What about trails versus pavement?

A. Running is running is running. As I mentioned earlier, when you up the amount of physical activity in any sport or training, you increase the chance of an overuse injury. I've seen some nasty treadmill spills (okay, I've been involved in a few too) and plenty of turned ankles on curbs and sidewalks, plenty of trips on trails and far too many falls on perfectly flat, smooth pavement. It happens to all of us. Think of the number of times you've tripped for no reason walking down a hallway. When you run, each mile exposes you to another 1500 to 2000 potential missteps.

If you want to become a stronger runner on all conditions, it's important that you run on varying surfaces. Trails, sidewalks, roads, tracks, treadmills... they're all a great place to run and you shouldn't fear any of them. The key is to mix up your terrain as often as possible.

Q. I heard that running on concrete sidewalks is harder and the impact is worse for my knees and back than running on pavement, which is softer. Is that true?

A. This is pretty funny, and I had a running partner who insisted it was true. A quick Internet search back in 2007 proved him wrong, and I never had to hear about it again. The hardness of pavement roads and concrete sidewalks doesn't provide any difference in the impact on your body from footfalls on it. Now, the slightly rougher surface of some newer sidewalks may cause your shoes to wear out a little bit more quickly, but that's a totally different story. Plus most cars don't drive on the sidewalk, so I recommend running on them versus the side of the road. Most sidewalks are relatively flat, as they were designed for—get this—runners and walkers to use and keep off the roads, while roads are sloped to allow water to run off of the driving surface. Running on the shoulder of the road means you're on an uneven surface that will cause unbalanced posture in your run and even injuries.

Q. I missed a couple scheduled runs. Do I have to start over?

A. We all miss workouts. The most important thing is to get back on your program as soon as you can. Work, family, illness, travel, holidays, injuries and plenty of other forces are conspiring against your planned exercise. It happens! If you miss a week, start from where you were. If you miss more than that, keep moving back your workout the same amount of time you missed. At about two weeks you begin to lose some of the base fitness and running acumen that you've built up.

Q. Taper? What's that?

A. Ten to seven days before your race, you need to back off your distance and intensity to recover and prepare for a race. For longer distances like a marathon, the taper will begin with reduced mileage 14 days before the race and as little as a light two- to three-mile jog to keep loose in the three to four days leading up to race day. You'll see what I'm talking about with the taper in the programs starting on page 85.

Q. Can I run every day?

A. Eventually, yes—but you need to build up your endurance and strength first. Experienced runners who lace up every day will vary their workouts between tempo runs, intervals, hill work, easy runs and longer distances to keep their body and mind fresh. Too many intense workouts back to back can lead to burnout, overuse injuries and overtraining. Too much of a good thing is still too much, and trying to do excessive amounts too soon is a sure way to knock you off track with injury or boredom. In the progams in Part 3, I cover how to avoid some common pitfalls of overtraining and losing your momentum.

Before You Begin

Guess what? I'm going to tell you to get off your ass and go to the doctor before you start this program. How does right now work for you? Chances are, you're a 20-minute visit away from a clean bill of health. Even if the doc does find anything alarming, you're much better off catching it early than having it sneak up on you later.

My wife Kristen absolutely forbade me from training for Ironman Arizona in 2009 until after I received a doctor's sign-off, and I'm glad I did. Hundreds of hours running, biking and swimming would've been a foolish undertaking had I not had my ticker checked out first. Suck it up, make a call and go see your doc.

Want one more reason to go see a doctor before you start? She'll give you some encouragement in your new pursuit of fitness (or at least she should) and when you come back for your next visit she'll be able to say, "Wow, you look great!" and maybe even pat herself on the back for getting you to follow doctor's orders!

If I didn't yet make it perfectly clear: Always obtain clearance from a doctor that you're healthy enough to begin this or any other strenuous exercise regimen. Perform each exercise within your ability and always use proper form. Most of all, don't be stupid and try to do too much, too fast—that's a recipe for a pulled muscle, shin splints or a bout of DOMS that will knock you off track from completing the next workout.

Listen to Your Body

You should be able to tell when you're ready to begin a strength and conditioning program like this one by tuning in to your body. Take it easy and be smart about determining what's normal soreness from a workout and what's a nagging injury that you're aggravating. If you think it's the latter, take a few extra days off and see if the soreness passes. If it doesn't, you should see a medical professional.

You should expect to experience mild soreness and fatigue, especially when you're just getting started. The feeling of your muscles being "pumped" after a workout or a hard run and the fatigue of an exhausting workout are normal, as is the flush of warmth when finishing a challenging set of intervals. These are positive feelings.

On the other hand, any sharp pain, muscle spasm or numbness is a warning sign that you need to stop and not push yourself any harder. Some muscle groups may fatigue more quickly because they're undertrained or have been unused for a while. Your quads, glutes, hips and calves are doing a tremendous amount of work and can easily fatigue. Your joints and feet are taking a lot more of a workload than they're used to and will surely become sore. If you feel uncomfortable and can't run anymore, walk. If you're really beat, light-headed or dizzy, stop immediately and rest. Get medical attention immediately if those symptoms persist or you feel any of these heart attack symptoms:

- Discomfort, pressure, heaviness or pain in the chest, arm or below the breastbone

- Discomfort radiating to the back, jaw, throat or arm

- Fullness, indigestion or a choking feeling (may feel like heartburn)

ANTI-INFLAMMATORIES

It's been said that "ibuprofen is a runner's best friend," but it's extremely easy to become too reliant on "vitamin I," causing health issues and even slowing your body's natural ability to heal. Inflammation is a normal part of the healing process when your cells essentially attack an "injured" area by increasing blood flow to speed up recovery. The swelling and pain associated with inflammation aids in healing, but also exacerbates the discomfort.

During training, performing the exercises creates small micro-tears in your muscles. When running, it happens with every single step you take. The harder or longer you run, the more stress is put on your muscles and the more micro-tears you'll have. While a muscle tear sounds like a bad thing, these micro-tears are actually good, as they help your muscles to strengthen and grow as they heal. The inflammatory response that's signaled by this muscle damage causes your body to deliver more blood, oxygen and nutrients to immediately begin the healing process. An anti-inflammatory (non-steroidal anti-inflammatory drug, or NSAIDs) can actually impede some of this rapid healing. Furthermore, an over-the-counter anti-inflammatory can mask some of the symptoms of more acute muscle strain or pain that could be signaling you to stop working out because there's some damage. You can't listen to your body if you're trying to get it to shut up and stop nagging you!

NSAIDs do have a positive role in reducing pain for short periods of time if you experience something like a low-grade sprain or somewhat sharp joint pain. With any severe pain, see a doctor immediately. Stop training and rest for one to three days while following the prescribed dose on the NSAID's bottle. After three days, reduce the dosage and let your body heal itself. Relying on an anti-inflammatory long-term can prevent you from healing and also potentially damage your kidneys if taken in prolonged heavy doses. If you have any questions, call your doctor.

- Sweating, nausea, vomiting or dizziness

- Extreme weakness, anxiety or shortness of breath

- Rapid or irregular heartbeats

Overtraining

The easiest way to spot overtraining is when you've trained successfully for a while and suddenly your results start to drop along with your energy and desire to keep on training. Guess what: This is your body telling you to stop! Too much of a good thing is still too much, and overtraining can quickly unravel all the gains you've gotten out of your efforts over the past few months.

Put simply, overtraining is training too hard and not allowing physical and mental recovery between workouts. The symptoms manifest as physical, behavioral and emotional stress that limits the athlete's ability to make progress, and can begin to diminish any strength and fitness gains they've made. While it's normally problematic in weight training, by incorporating cross-training and intense intervals it's common in runners and athletes of all types as well. Too much of a good thing is a bad thing—you can absolutely run and train too much to your own detriment!

Overtraining may be accompanied by one or more concomitant symptoms:

- Persistent muscle soreness and fatigue

- Elevated resting heart rate and reduced heart rate variability

- Increased incidence of injuries

- Irritability

- Depression

- Irregular sleep patterns

- Mental breakdown

This goes to show that overtraining is nothing to be trifled with, and the best way to combat it is by lowering your training volume or upping your rest and recovery time. Check out "Rest, the Secret Weapon" on page 73.

Here's my secret formula for preventing overtraining and maximizing recovery (okay, so it's not much of a secret):

RUN > REFUEL > RECOVER > REST > REPEAT

Run (or work out) 3 to 5 days a week based on your physical ability and previous conditioning. Beginners should take every other day off or put in a relatively light effort while more advanced athletes can mix in one or two "off-days" per week.

Refuel immediately after a hard workout lasting more than 30 minutes with a drink that contains a 4:1 carb-to-protein ratio. The carbs help to replace the glycogen you burned off for energy while also shuttling the protein to your muscles to speed recovery.

Recover with post-workout stretching, foam rolling, an ice bath (if you're brave), a trip to a steam room, a dip in a whirlpool or a warm tub with some dissolved Epsom salts, by slipping on some compression socks, or even getting a full-body deep-tissue massage. I can only personally vouch for the post-workout stretching, foam rolling, and deep-tissue massage as being extremely beneficial to a faster recovery, but I'll never pass up a chance to sit in the hot tub! The jury is still out on compression socks, so try them for yourself if you're interested. Personally, I'm a fan although I can't say it's any more effective than a placebo.

Rest for at least 8 hours a night, and be sure to use your off-days as off-days—not time to sneak in additional workouts! Get tips that pro athletes use for developing good rest habits on page 74.

Repeat as necessary. You can't stick with a program unless you keep at it until it becomes second nature. By maximizing your rest and recovery, you also greatly increase the odds that you'll be ready, willing and eager to tackle your next workout.

Gear

Okay, I'll admit it: I'm a gear geek. When I was first getting into running, I drove my running partners totally nuts by talking incessantly about the newest gizmos until I finally bought each of them. I then continued to play with them or rave about how amazing they were until my friends just started ignoring me any time I started a sentence with, "Hey, have you seen the new...?" Watches, heart monitors, running belts, sunglasses, tops, shorts, socks—I felt that everything could be improved through technology, especially shoes.

My collection of the latest and greatest shoes grew to include at least one pair from each major manufacturer and plenty from specialty shops that most non-runners have never heard of. I've logged miles in so many different shoes, at one point I could practically recite all the differences between models and brands better than a shoe salesman. Eventually, in order to keep my wife from killing me, I settled on a few models from one or two of my favorite brands for road or trail running. I'm lucky enough to test some incredibly high-tech shoes before they even hit the shelves due to my partnership with a rather innovative manufacturer, so I get my geek fix several times a year.

So that's how I am with technology, but it doesn't have to be the way you roll. Many of my training partners get discounts on last year's models and could care less about having the latest gizmos to track their workouts—they just want to enjoy their run.

Finding the Right Shoes

At the end of the day, you can do without any other high-tech toys just as long as you have the proper shoes for running style, surface and biomechanics. When it comes to shoes, one type does not suit all runners. I recommend you go to a full-service running store that offers professional video gait analysis so you can get fitted in the proper shoes. Below is just a guideline based solely (shoe pun intended) on the rough description of pronation and

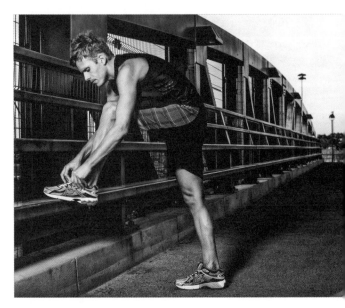

footprint. Get fitted by a professional or you may end up with a lighter wallet and painful shoes.

The portion of each stride where your foot is in contact with the ground is called the stance phase. During this time, a force two to three times your body weight is being placed on that foot and radiating up successive body parts (sing·along: "...the ankle bone's connected to the shin bone..."). As your body moves over your foot, it will transition from initial contact to toe-off with your heel turning inward toward your body's midline. This is called pronation, which is essential for stabilizing your body during the stance phase.

About 15 degrees is considered normal "rolling" of the foot to absorb the impact when running, ending with the runner pushing off evenly from all toes. Normal (or neutral) pronators make up about 15 percent of all runners, although there are many shades of "slightly over- or underpronators" that could easily fit into this group. Neutral runners will commonly have a normal arch to their foot; when stepping out of the shower their footprint looks like there's a missing imprint area where about 45% of their midfoot doesn't touch the floor.

Normal pronation shoe types: Neutral shoes, cushioned models, minimalist shoes and lightweight racers

Overpronation occurs when the foot makes contact with the ground and the heel rotates more than the standard 15 degrees. Due to this the toe-off is limited to just the big toe. The foot and ankle have to work hard to stabilize the body, hence the advent of stability shoes. When running behind an over-pronator, you'll notice the ankle is pointed inward at impact. If this describes you, don't fret. Overpronators make up about 75% of runners. Usually associated with flat feet, an overpronator will leave a wet footprint that has the entire surface of the foot touching the ground.

Overpronation shoe types: Stability-specific shoes or neutral, cushioned, minimalist and even lightweight racers that have some additional support

Underpronation is the opposite of overpronation (wow, big surprise!) in that the heel rotates less than 15 degrees at impact, and the foot rolls toward your little toe at toe-off. Once again, the ankle and foot have to work hard to keep your body under control. You can spot the somewhat rare underpronator by their ankle pointing outward as their foot makes impact. The footprint of a severe overpronator will show an unusually high arch, even so much as to

have a gap all the way from the lateral to medial side of the foot.

Underpronation shoe types: Motion-control shoes or neutral, cushioned and some minimalist shoes with motion control inserts

After all that talk of pronation, there's another school of thought that you can wear whatever shoe you'd like and see if it works for you. I'm an overpronator who wears racing flats almost exclusively with no problems at all. Sometimes you need to know the rules before you break them!

REPLACING AND ROTATING YOUR SHOES

Over time, the foam and other space-age materials in your fancy-schmancy new shoes will break down and the tread will wear out. In order for there to be a multi-billion-dollar shoe market, you need to buy new shoes. While there's no magic number, 400 miles or about six months of normal running seems to be the rough amount of time before runners toss their busted-up kicks and pick up a new pair. I have a few pairs that have lasted long after this loosely established expiration date, and every so often I'll take them out for a run when I want to change things

> "Swap out your training shoes for running 'flats' [lighter-weight racing shoes] for race day. Your feet will feel light and you'll feel faster, like you traded in your VW for a Ferrarri."
> —Lewis Elliot, professional triathlete, U.S. National Cycling champion

up a bit and rotate through different shoes. By swapping out different pairs from one run to the next you can avoid some common issues, like hot spots or blisters, and allow the foam in your shoes to recover from the constant beating they take cushioning 1500 to 2000 foot strikes per mile. I'll still pick up a new pair every three months but I'll rotate it with a pair that's only essentially been used for a month and a half, and can easily tell the difference when the old shoe's cushioning is nearing the end of its life.

Clothing

When picking out clothing for all temperatures and conditions, the most important thing is that it fits well, is comfortable and allows full range of motion. No matter how pretty that new running top may be, if it causes irritation on the inside of your arm each time you swing it, you'll be miserable by the end of your run. There are millions of choices for clothing in all varieties of high-tech material to chose from, but the bottom line is being comfortable.

TIP: Don't wear that race's T-shirt at that race—unless it's famous for it. Pat's Run in Tempe, Arizona, is one of those races, with nearly every one of the 20,000 participants proudly wearing "42" in honor of Pat Tillman. Pat's Run changes the color and design every year, so each race is run with a sea of 42s in different colors from participants of previous years.

A great pair of comfortable running shorts can last a long time, so don't be afraid to spend a little extra on a few pairs that have the right pockets you may want for training and a pair or two just for racing. Remember, comfort is not optional, and chafing is the enemy. If the shorts you're running in are uncomfortable, they are NOT good running shorts, no matter what the label says. Don't be afraid to ditch a pair of trendy shorts or demote them to being worn around the house if they don't remain comfortable throughout your runs.

Shirts are another matter altogether. Unless you're a big fan of sleeveless running singlets, most T-shirts will do as long as they're a blend of some sort. One hundred percent cotton will soak with sweat and either get clingy and uncomfortable or baggy and uncomfortable as you work out hard. Either way, it's no *bueno*. The good news: Most running races provide T-shirts and, with prices on tech material on the decline, you'll usually get a poly-cotton blend or even a moisture-wicking style. I haven't purchased a running shirt in an extremely long time, and have dozens of new and semi-worn shorts from events in my closet.

Socks are extremely important, and the wrong choice can end a training day or race with a blister rather easily. Unfortunately, no one can tell you ahead of time what sock/shoe combination will cause issues, and you'll need to test out a few different solutions for yourself. As with shirts, 100% cotton socks are a bad idea when sweat is involved! There are many types of socks featuring multiple layers, high-tech anti-friction material, compression to prevent your feet from swelling up and even some with little pockets for each toe to prevent chafing between your little piggies. Whatever you try, make sure you test your socks out on a medium to long run before you ever decide to wear them on race day. You should never race in clothes or shoes that you've never tested before!

Anti-chafing cream or spray works wonders on limiting discomfort and preventing blisters or hot spots on areas where skin can potentially get rubbed raw. The lateral area on your torso just below your armpits is a common area for skin irritation when the inside of your arm rubs, as are the insides of your thighs, nipples and even between your butt cheeks! Anywhere there's a rub, there will potentially be discomfort or even a blister. Anti-chafe works very well on feet to prevent hot spots with new shoes or socks, especially during the break-in period. Before long training runs or races, I'll often apply anti-chafe at the same time I put on sunscreen.

Music, Gizmos & Other Gear

From reading articles on many of my favorite running blogs and magazine sites, it seems to be the consensus that most runners enjoy training and racing while cranking some tunes through their ear buds. Running with music can help to erase the doldrums and the monotony of training and motivate you when you need a push. Music can also distract you while training and is often responsible for runners not hearing other people, cyclists or even vehicles coming up behind them. In order to keep us all safe out there, let's agree to the following rough guidelines:

Treadmill: Volume 80–100%—Crank it as high as you want to drown out the bad gym tunes and the sound of the guy panting next to you. In the gym, earphones are the universal symbol for "I'm here to exercise, don't bother me" and will hopefully keep someone from distracting you with questions about changing the TV station or how to use the elliptical machine.

Trail & Sidewalk: Volume 60–70%— Metallica is pumping through your cranium, but you can hear other bikers, runners, dogs or even horses coming up from behind. If you haven't been passed by a wild burro on a trail, consider yourself (and your underpants) lucky—it's like being too close to a freight train that's gone off the tracks. Keeping your volume low enough that you can hear a biker yelling "on your left" or "heads up" is crucial, and also keeping the tunes low enough so you can hear a car backing out of a blind driveway or other runners' footsteps when they're close will save you from being startled at the last second and give you plenty of time to react. It's tough to continue running when your heart leaps from your chest, right? When on sidewalks, always make eye contact with every driver possible in cars at intersections before crossing.

Road: Volume 10–50%—Keep your tunes as low as possible so that you can hear your favorite track and still be aware of everything—and I mean everything—that's going on around you. All kidding aside, runners are completely, entirely vulnerable when on the roads no matter how far away from the main city streets they are. In a situation where a driver doesn't see you, it's up to you to get out of the way. There's no "right" or "wrong" to worry about when a two-ton block of steel is hurtling into your path, and absolutely no honor in standing your ground if this happens. Be smart, be safe and be 100% aware of your surroundings when you run anywhere near vehicles or roadways. Some more tips on running safely can be found in "Getting Started" on page 40.

Race: Volume 0%—Leave your tunes at home. The official sanctioning body for all standardized races in the United States, USA Track & Field (USATF), forbids them for all championships and runners competing for medals, awards or prize money in their events. Now, if that doesn't pertain to you, wearing headphones is allowed, but I still strongly recommend against it. Even on courses closed to traffic, there are still many situations when runner safety is compromised by loud music: volunteers or emergency crew members giving safety direction on the course in the case of an injured runner or any on-course danger ahead, police or emergency vehicles needing to cross the course, faster runners alerting you that they're passing on your left or right so you don't step in front of them, just to name

a few. The bottom line is: You need to be aware of your surroundings when you're running along with hundreds, thousands or even tens of thousands of other runners. Plugging your ears isn't necessarily a smart move.

You may also be missing out on the sounds of the cheering crowd or other runners saying hi or "nice run" while passing or pacing with you. During the hectic water stops, it's a good idea to know if there's someone directly behind you and to be aware of your surroundings; in-ear music can easily be a distraction. Trust me, there's plenty of worthwhile distractions like live bands, cowbells, DJs and more out on the course!

In addition, when you race with music, you miss out on the social experience, or even miss out on the race all together! Tricia Schafer, a Phoenix runner who has competed in more than 100 races in the past five years, initially raced with music to combat anxiety, but finally ditched the tunes in mid-2009. "And I'm glad I did! In 2008 I passed some friendly rivals in a challenging 10K, only to make a wrong turn and lose my lead. Because of my music, I couldn't hear race officials calling out to me to turn back. Now, instead of focusing on my tunes I enjoy hearing cheers from the sidelines and encouragement from other runners as they pass me on the course. Running without music actually changed my life. Two words I heard loud and clear, at mile 2 of a 5K in 2010: 'You're fast!' All I could muster in response was a grunt, as the man who uttered them sprinted ahead. I chased him to the finish, a mere 11 seconds behind—my 5K PR to this day. And I never let him go. The man? Johnny Lookabaugh, who is now my partner in business and in life."

I've been lucky enough to run some amazing races in unbelievably beautiful areas all over the United States—from sea to shining sea, plains to mountains—with and without tunes. Sometimes you need to pull your earphones out just to soak in all the majesty of the incredible scenery. In nearly every race I've run, from 5Ks to ultramarathons, the quick words or conversations I've had with friends and even total strangers have been more valuable to me than hearing the same searing guitar riffs that I've heard thousands of times over the years. I've taken to eschewing the iPod and I'm even more thankful for the chance to interact with others who share the same passion for running. On that note, remember to say hi, raise your hand in a slight wave, smile or nod back when another runner makes eye contact. Be polite and courteous whether you have earphones in or not; it's a simple gesture that goes a long way when training or racing and we all appreciate it. No one's asking you to chat up all 30,000 other racers at a marathon corral—just don't be a wet blanket. Running karma can be fickle; be on the safe side by being friendly to other runners.

Gadgets go much further than a simple music player and include myriad devices and smartphone apps that can track just about every metric that you can think of. Some of them even track you while you sleep! If you're the type of runner who likes data on every single workout or run, there's no shortage of ways for you to find a gizmo or app to give you all the metrics you're looking for.

I've already come clean that I'm a certifiable tech junkie, so it should come as no surprise that I've tested out a bunch of these devices over the years and even specifically requested some while testing the programs for this book. You can check out my updated gear guide on www.7weekstofitness.com/gear to see some of my long-standing favorites and newest hot toys to play with during (and between) my runs.

With the help of Chris, one of my favorite tech geeks (and I mean that as an absolute term of endearment), we developed our own smartphone app for the *7 Weeks to a 10K* programs. You can take your workouts along with you and use it to keep track of your training. It's available with the apps from some of my other books at www.7weekstofitness.com/products/app.

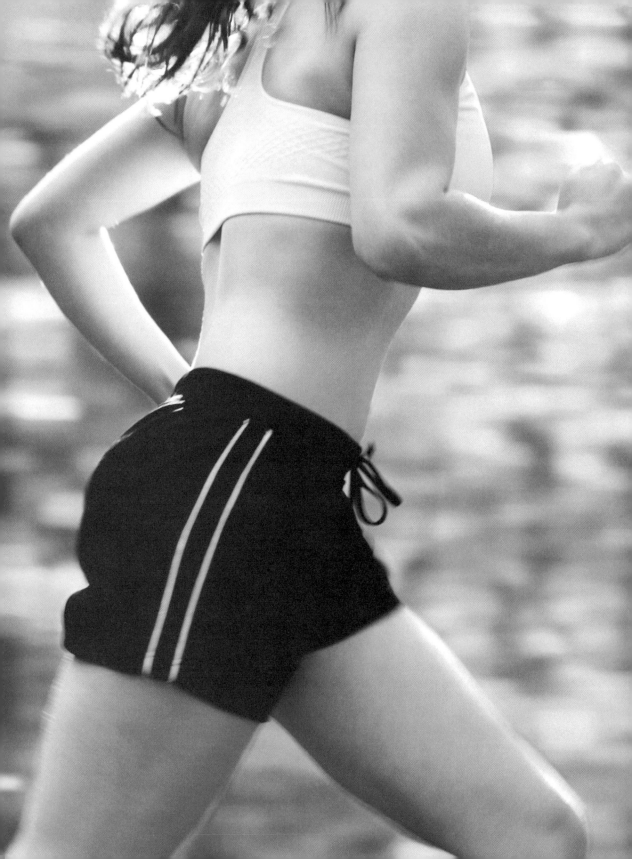

PART 2:
RUNNING 101

Getting Started

"The best time to plant a tree was 20 years ago. The second best time is now."
—*CHINESE PROVERB*

Running is a commitment of time, physical energy and mental energy, but it's far more important than a simple pastime to pick up. A fitness and running regimen is an investment that you make in yourself, and the potential dividends are many: a healthier, happier life; a sense of accomplishment by reaching your goals; the fortitude that comes from learning from mistakes and fighting through setbacks to keep your goals in sight.

There will be many ups and downs during your running career, and you'll learn valuable lessons from each victory and many more from any failures and stumbles along the way to hit your goals. Some training sessions will feel like a trip to the dentist while others will feel like a day at the spa. To adopt a runner's mentality means to embrace the good with the bad and keep an open mind to all the things you'll learn along the way. I personally never envisioned becoming a runner. I cherish all the memories I've made "on the run" and look forward to the experiences I've yet to have.

So, how does one get started and become a runner? It all starts with a simple desire to reach a goal, whether it's to run a marathon, lose weight, feel better, change your life or even just get off the couch and do something. Harnessing that desire can be a tricky thing— just think of the millions of New Year's resolutions that fall by the wayside mere minutes or days after they've been made. True aspirations still need to be combined with a plan of action in order to make them a reality, and continued repetition is required to make that action into a routine.

Here are some simple tips and recommendations in order to make a plan and stick with it, to become a runner for the first time or to develop better running habits that can lead to an even more successful and enjoyable running career.

START SMALL. No one becomes an athlete overnight. It takes time to build up your strength, skill and stamina. Begin by walking and jogging short distances and stick with it. You'll soon be going farther and faster than you ever expected. Give yourself the chance to progress and your body to adapt.

WALK BEFORE YOU RUN. walk/ jog intervals are a big part of the Prep Program (page 88) and should absolutely be the path for new runners to build up their strength and stamina before running any continuous amount. The short walking breaks will allow you to catch your breath, hydrate and prepare to execute the next jog with a relaxed stride and proper form.

GO SHORT BEFORE YOU GO LONG. The quickest way for a new runner or one coming back after an injury to get knocked off track is to try and log too many miles, too fast. It's extremely common to get excited about completing an enjoyable run and immediately try to run significantly farther the next time you head out to train. Think of it like lifting weights: You don't jump from curling 10-pound dumbbells to suddenly lifting a pair of 35s the next day. It takes time to progressively build up your mileage the same way. Failing to take your time will result in sore joints, shin splints, "dead" legs that have little energy and no spring in them, and delayed onset muscle soreness (DOMS). Any of these injuries can knock you off track for your training, and all are easily avoidable by progressively adding to your mileage in small increments over time. The Prep Program was designed specifically for newcomers to start from scratch and get into running. For semi-experienced runners, a common rule of thumb is to add 10% to your mileage each week, but I like to use a simpler method: Pick one run per week and add a mile to it. Repeat each week until you get to your target distance. Adding mileage doesn't go on forever!

Below is an example of adding mileage similar to what we'll see in all the programs. This is also an effective and safe way for experienced runners to increase their endurance and strength (aka "base") when stepping up to a longer race distance or coming back from off-season or injury. The Prep Program (page 88) starts with progressive walking and jogging intervals based on time, while the Basic and Level 2 Programs use progressive distance additions. (Check out "Preparing for the Programs" on page 75 for a primer on intervals and progression.)

Week 1 Monday: 3 miles
Wednesday: 3 miles
Friday: 3 miles
total: 9 miles

Week 2 Monday: 4 miles
Wednesday: 3 miles
Friday: 3 miles
total: 10 miles

Week 3 Monday: 4 miles
Wednesday: 4 miles
Friday: 3 miles
total: 11 miles

Week 4 Monday: 4 miles
Wednesday: 4 miles
Friday: 4 miles
total: 12 miles

Progressive programs with an incremental gain can work wonders over time. Just try and hold yourself back from jumping into longer distances too quickly.

GO SLOW BEFORE YOU GO FAST. Speed, like distance, also takes time to build up to as it's extremely easy to damage muscle tissue that's not yet conditioned for rapid bursts of speed, and the injuries can be quite catastrophic in nature. Severe muscle or tendon pulls and tears can happen in an instant and take weeks, months or years to heal, if they do. Sprinting only takes place in the Level 2 Program and for finite periods of time.

RUN WITH A PAL (TWO- OR FOUR-LEGGED VARIETY). If you already have a pooch and are a beginner, then you have a training partner. The walk/jog intervals are perfect for giving both you and your dog a boost in your daily routine. The short-distance jogs are a great way to begin to build your cardio and base mileage, and probably won't completely wear either of you out too quickly. Knowing your doggie needs you to take her out anyway makes it easier to sneak this workout into your normal day, and I'm pretty positive Fido will enjoy it. You'll both get fitter together and mutually build up your distance between walks. I run with my pooch all the time; check out "What Shelby Taught Me about Pacing" (page 80).

Humans happen to make pretty darn good running partners too. They usually complain a little more than your dog does, but at least they don't try and trip you with

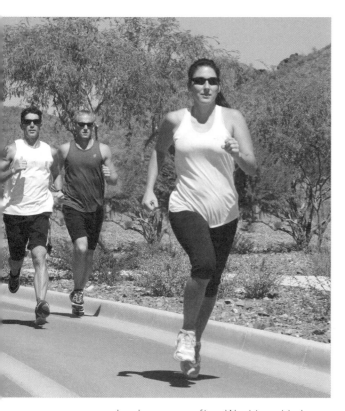

sluggish, slow to your pace when you're not feeling well and stay with you when you need a rest. The key is to make sure you both support each other along the way. The "Golden Rule" applies to runners: Make sure you help out your partner as you'd like them to help you out!

As you and your partner get more experienced as runners, invariably you'll start to push and challenge each other, but keep this in check. Each training run shouldn't be required to end with a sprint—unless that's what you're both up for. When training back at ESPN with my partners Erik and Mandy, all three of us were so close in our pace that each run we'd have a different "winner." Head-to-head sprints to the finish are commonplace every time I run with Michael Bennett here in the desert. Two ultra-competitive guys trying to push each other on every single workout can be a fantastic thing!

RUN FAST, THINK FAST.

Studies have shown that physical exercise helps brain cell development and neural connections; researchers are attributing this to increased oxygen and nutrient flow during cardiovascular exercise. In other words, the more you run, the more you strengthen your mind too! The thought process of most runners will fall into three categories:

Thinking about running while running. This group is usually composed of new runners who haven't yet learned to relax and let the training run happen. Incidentally, this also happens to be the

a leash every so often. Want to get to know someone? Go for a run with them! Running works just like truth serum; after a mile or so complete strangers will tell you just about anything about their life. It must have something to do with all the endorphins swirling around your brain, and you can't help it. Also, by the end of a good run, you'll end up being better friends with your running partner too.

The mere existence of a running partner will usually be enough to get you out of bed on a cold, dim morning to head out for a run so you don't let them down. Optimally, one of you should be a morning person—that's a big help! A good running partner will motivate you when you're same group that complains how much running sucks.

Thinking about absolutely nothing—completely "out of it" while running. I happen to know a few of these types who can literally shut off their brain and just chug through the miles. From my experience, these are the runners who you need to be extremely careful when running with on a busy street as they have a tendency to completely forget about road or sidewalk conditions, car, pedestrian or bike traffic and even dog poo. Like Forrest Gump said: "It happens!"

Thinking about anything and everything else while running: exploring the meaning of life and the existential nature of beings one minute and then contemplating who gave the paperclip its shape and why Benjamin Franklin would choose a wild turkey for the national bird of the United States. I happen to fall into this category, and find that during a run I'm in the perfect mental space to think about writing, projects and all sorts of creative endeavors.

LOSE WEIGHT WHILE RUNNING, BUT DON'T RUN TO LOSE WEIGHT. As a coach and trainer, "I want to lose X pounds by Y date" is one of the most common phrases I'll hear, and while it's a lofty and admirable goal, it's fraught with problems. Running is a great way to lose weight, but it's not the end-all-be-all of fitness, especially for those who are overweight and can't yet take full advantage of the cardiovascular and metabolic benefits due

to the additional force placed on joints and a limited aerobic capacity. Aside from the physical conditioning, weight loss is dependent on proper nutrition and caloric intake. Running will not make you thin if your diet does not support healthy weight loss.

Setting too short of a time frame for losing weight is also snafu that can lead to depression, low self-esteem and even extremely unhealthy methods to drop pounds by using fat-burning pills, diuretics, laxatives or worse. Trying to lose too much, too fast is a sure way to miss your goal.

Now, don't let me deter you from employing a running regimen to get in shape and lose weight. Running is one of the most efficient ways to burn calories—a whopping 100 or so per mile for a 150-pound person at a 9:30-per-mile pace. There's no doubt you can get stronger, fitter and torch the fat off your body by sticking with a running plan, but combining it with proper nutrition and a full-body exercise regimen will give you the results you're seeking much faster. (Read all about it in "The Programs" on page 85.) The Achilles heel to weight loss for most new runners comes from overestimating the amount of calories they burned while running and taking in too many calories as a result.

Here's a little cheat sheet to give you an idea what your calorie burn is really like so you can think twice before "treating yourself" to a celebratory doughnut after your workout. Calculations are based on the amount of calories a 150-pound man can expect to burn in 1 hour:

> "Save your energy. All that extra stuff you're doing with your arms and hands just drains your juice. Control your motion—run like a robot or that guy from *Terminator 2*."
> —Scot Little, elite amateur triathlete

- Sedentary, little or no exercise: BMR x 1.2

- Light exercise or sports 1–3 days per week: BMR x 1.375

- Moderate exercise or sports 3–5 days per week: BMR x 1.55

- Hard exercise or sports 6–7 days per week: BMR x 1.725

- Very hard exercise, amateur to professional athlete: BMR x 1.9

Running @ 10:00 pace: ~700 calories
Running @ 19:00 pace: ~230
Sitting on couch: ~100

The last one may throw you for a loop. You would've burned about 100 calories by sitting on your butt and letting your body's systems do their thing. Your BMR, or Basal Metabolic Rate, is essentially the amount of calories your body would burn if you stayed in bed all day long, and it's probably higher than you think. I was personally astonished to learn that mine was over 1600, and then used it as a tool to calculate the number of calories I should take in per day to maintain my weight and support my bodily functions based on my physical activity.

BMR Formula for males:

BMR = 66 + (6.23 X WEIGHT IN POUNDS) + (12.7 X HEIGHT IN INCHES)–(6.8 X AGE IN YEARS)

For example, I'm 5'9" (69 inches), 155 pounds and 42 years of age; my BMR is 1622.35.

BMR Formula for females:

BMR = 655 + (4.35 X WEIGHT IN POUNDS) + (4.7 X HEIGHT IN INCHES)–(4.7 X AGE IN YEARS)

Caloric Intake (Harris Benedict Formula)

Based on your daily level of activity, multiply your BMR by the factor in the following table to get the number of calories you should consume in a day to maintain your weight and proper bodily functions.

With a BMR of 1622.35 and a multiplier of 1.725 during hard training, my caloric intake should be around 2800 calories per day.

If you're planning to use this BMR and caloric guidelines to lose weight, don't go overboard. Reducing your intake by 500 calories a day is a substantial amount and a good guideline to go by for healthy weight loss when combined with light to moderate exercise. If you plan on upping the intensity, keep your calories right around the calculated number above and you should lose weight effectively as well. Learn more about losing weight while training on "Dropping Weight to Begin Running" in the Prep Program on page 89.

RUN FOR SOMEONE ELSE.
Running for a charity or in honor of someone who can no longer run for themselves is a way to tap into a whole other well of strength in order to keep going. If your mantra becomes "I won't quit on Pat Tillman," then it may be much easier to train for Pat's Run while also

raising money for the Tillman Foundation. I'm proud to be a member of Team Tillman, and the process of raising funds while training for one of Arizona's biggest marathons kept me motivated. During my training for Ironman in 2009, I covered my bike with names of friends and family who had fought cancer and enlisted the help of others to help me reach my financial goal to donate to the Prostate Cancer Foundation. During any low times during training or the race when I thought about quitting or even dropping out due to a flat tire (it happens!), I remembered each one of those courageous individuals and it was a no-brainer to tough it out till the end.

Through progressive training, the incremental improvements you make over time will add up to very significant gains. My first race was 3.1 miles, my last race was over 50, but it doesn't happen overnight. I'll show you in "The Programs" on page 85 how to make every workout count and build on the last effort to make you faster, fitter and stronger. Through repetition over time, you'll continue to build your endurance and progress even farther as a runner. The sky's the limit, but you'll need to put in some time and hard work before you can go "swinging on a star."

COME BACK ALIVE—RUN SAFELY.

Running isn't all that dangerous. Compared to any other physical sport, the incidents that result in serious injury are minimal, but unless you're confined to running only on a treadmill, there are dangerous environmental and situational factors that need to be kept in mind. I've put together a whole section about runner safety (see page 47) with plenty of things to be aware of and tactics to keep you safe. Most importantly, use common sense when running and avoid potentially unsafe conditions and situations; whenever possible, run with a friend and always carry a cell phone when you're out alone.

Running Safely

Heart attacks, collisions with cars and falls from trails are responsible for the majority of runners' deaths. Throw in the serious injuries caused by wild animals and extreme temperatures and there are plenty of conditions you should be aware of while on the run.

Undiagnosed heart conditions can, and have, fallen the best of runners and some of the most otherwise healthy and fit individuals on the planet. Remember when I asked you to go see a doctor BEFORE starting this program? Well, you made an appointment, right? What you don't know CAN hurt you when it comes to an unhealthy heart, especially when you'll be exerting yourself while training and racing. Please—take a few minutes to make an appointment and show up. Also, on page 28 I covered the signs of a heart attack. From different reports I've read, you may be well-served to always bring an aspirin along with you on your runs; it could save your life. If you have a history of any heart ailments, let your running partner know. In the event of any sort of sharp chest pain or dizziness, stop running immediately and attempt to catch your breath. If you experience any symptoms of a heart attack, ask your partner to dial 911.

As a pedestrian, you're usually within your rights to walk, run or jog just about anywhere on public property, but when it comes to a showdown between two tons of steel and a human, the advantage is clearly not in your favor. Just because a vehicle is supposed to stop and let you cross or at least give a cursory pause at a stop sign doesn't mean it will. I've personally been tossed over the hood of a pick-up truck that didn't stop at an intersection, luckily avoiding any serious harm.

This book is dedicated to the memory of one of the finest marathoners and triathletes hailing from the American Southwest, Sally Meyerhoff, whose talent and personality was taken away from the running community due to a training collision with an automobile. If this loss can teach us anything, it's always to be aware of your surroundings when sharing the road with vehicles and to always err on the side of caution when dealing with drivers who may be distracted or just not see you.

As a runner on the roadways who wishes to remain safe, it becomes your job to make sure you're seen by every vehicle—including bikes. This includes being in the right place, acting in a predictable manner, obeying traffic signals, wearing bright or easily noticeable clothing, using lights and reflective apparel at night and being hyperaware of every vehicle around you.

Where to Safely Run

Sidewalks and trails are by far the safest places for runners to avoid contact with motorized vehicles, and should be chosen over a road for safety's sake whenever they're present. Many forward-thinking states have adopted programs to turn unused train tracks into pedestrian zones, sometimes called linear parks, prairie paths, rails-to-trails or some other friendly name; these areas are your best bet to run safely without much concern for cars except at road crossings. Bikes, rollerblades and skateboarders may be a bit of a nuisance and there's some potential for a painful collision, so always keep aware of your surroundings, run toward the right of the path and allow faster individuals to pass. If you're listening to tunes, keep it at a reasonable volume so you can hear someone coming up from behind you, hopefully alerting you that they're about to pass you by shouting out a quick "on your left!"

Sidewalks sometimes get a bad rap as they can be uneven around joints, canted at the end of driveways, have more curves than a road, and a list of other relatively inconsequential reasons why "serious" runners prefer to run on the road. Personally, I've heard many excuses to run on the road. Here are a couple of my favorites:

- *"Sidewalks are harder than pavement and therefore cause shin splints."* This is complete bunk; the impact of a footfall on a sidewalk is no more damaging than one on pavement. Actually, roads are crowned to help water run-off so you're doing more damage to your hips, ankles, knees and IT bands by running on a

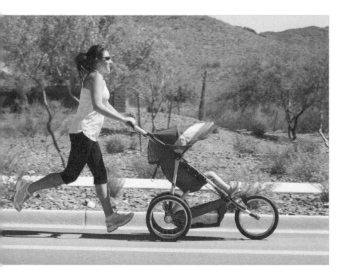

road's sloped surface than you would on sidewalks that were made specifically for pedestrians.

- *"Marathons aren't held on sidewalks so why would I want to train on them?"* Marathons also aren't held on roads that are open to traffic, right? Any idiot that would make this argument should go out and run any big-city marathon course during the week, preferably around rush hour.

Sidewalks are not without their fair share of dangers: vehicles backing out of driveways, aggressive dogs, cracks and potholes, muggers, low-handing branches and maybe even the occasional lemonade stand. Be aware of your surroundings. Be prepared to dodge obstacles and stay safe.

If you must run on the road, always do it facing traffic. Always—even on quiet neighborhood streets. For one, you can always see the traffic that's closest to you and attempt to make eye contact with the driver to make sure they see you and also move farther off the road to give a wide berth for the occasional vehicle that strays too far toward the edge of the road. There are even some drivers that aim to scare runners or even worse; keeping oncoming traffic in front of you affords you more time to react if you need to get out of the way. Walk and run against traffic, bike with it—keeping with this predictable pattern makes it simpler for pedestrians, cyclists and vehicles to coexist.

Keeping with the term "predictability," always make your movements in and around traffic consistent; quickly darting in a tangent out in front of vehicles isn't safe for anyone. Even if you aren't hit, you can cause a chain reaction that causes accidents or hurts others. You may also be culpable for a deeper injury to runners the world over—acting like an asshole that causes drivers to hate runners, and in turn take aggressive actions against them in the future. If you don't think this sentiment exists, I hate to inform you that you're wrong. There are plenty of motorists that despise sharing the road with runners and cyclists, and it only takes one altercation with or perceived slight by a runner to give agitated drivers a "reason" for a vendetta against other innocent runners or cyclists.

FALLS ON OR FROM TRAILS

Trails are a great surface for mixing up your training. The varying terrain and hills will help strengthen supporting muscles as well as kick your workout up a notch in intensity as well as provide some new scenery instead of the same old roads. Of course, with varying terrain on dirt trails, you have rocks, roots, branches, flora and fauna, cacti (hey, I'm from Arizona!) and wildlife to deal with. Horses, mountain bikers, and hikers usually will be using the same trails, so it's important you're aware of your fellow outdoor enthusiasts as well.

Trips and falls are commonly worse on trails than they would be on a sidewalk or road. The uneven surfaces can easily catch your foot and most trail surfaces aren't conducive to a fall without some scrapes and bruises—and that's in the relatively controlled falls where you stay on the trail. In steeper terrain, trails can be narrow and treacherous, and often a trip can lead to a long, steep fall down a hill into rocks, trees or the aforementioned cacti. In any situation, falling from a trail is an extremely bad thing, so never run alone on a remote and tricky trail and always take it slowly over treacherous, steep terrain. In sketchy, technical or difficult areas, make sure to maintain stable footing on rocks or loose dirt and lift your feet up to avoid stubbing your toes, resulting in a stumble. Keep your steps short and light, and always tackle difficult terrain with a partner and with plenty of daylight. Never forget: You can walk dangerous sections of any trail if you don't feel comfortable. Be careful, smart and stay safe.

Aggressive Dogs

I love my dog; she's a fun running partner and a goofy pup with a sweet disposition. Because Shelby's a bull terrier and a muscular dog with a solid stance, many other runners will cross a road or avoid us when we're out for a run, and I think that's the best course of action. When you meet a dog at a park, there's a good chance you're seeing the positive attributes of that pup; when you're running by or startle a dog from behind, even the most well-trained canine will be a little bit spooked and react with anything from a quick glance to a jump in your direction.

As a race director, I personally witnessed one of my racers get bit by a dog that another competitor brought along with him. This well-trained pooch was on a leash and running right along with its owner and was startled by a fellow competitor passing and lunged at her leg. Luckily, the passing runner wasn't hurt badly, but it could've been much, much worse for everyone if she had been.

Remember, you're out for a run and, unless you're Barry Siff (a famous athlete, coach and race director who just can't help himself but to stop and pet every dog he sees), you don't need to be stopping for a pooch break. For the record, some other owners may not like it all that much anyway. When I'm out for a run with Shelby, I surely don't want to be stopped no matter how excited she is to see someone new.

Give any dog and owner a wide berth when you're running toward them and cross the road if you can or at least slow down enough to provide the owner an opportunity to place them between you and the dog. If you're approaching from behind, give a little shout ahead to alert the owner that you're on your way and then follow the earlier directions: Give plenty of room, stay out of lunging reach based on the length of the leash and allow the owner to place the dog on the opposite side of them away from you. If you can cross the road easily and safely to avoid unnecessary dog confrontations, then go right ahead.

Unleashed, wild and aggressive dogs are not to be trifled with; wild animals can be unpredictable for a variety of different reasons. Hunger, injury, fear or abuse can be motivators for them to attack you if you're in the wrong place at the wrong time. Even a friendly pooch that has gotten lost can react aggressively due to being lost or scared. Always be alert when running, and scan areas ahead of you for any potential encounter. Keep your music low enough that you can hear a dog barking or snarling behind you; the simple act of you running may be fueling their hunter/prey instincts.

Avoid contact with unknown dogs. If you see a loose dog ahead, stop running and assess their behavior. If they're running toward you, act quickly and find a safe or defensive position. Look for an open door of a building or car; jump onto a parked car and scramble to the roof if necessary. The insurance claim is much better than the alternative. Do not run unless you can get to safety before the dog can catch you. Your flight will cause the dog to look at you as prey.

If the dog is holding its ground, stop and slowly walk backward or sideways, keeping the dog in your peripheral vision until the threat has passed. Do not run until the dog has lost its focus and interest in you. Stay calm and project that you're strong and in control of the situation. Your body language says a lot to a dog: Stand up straight and don't cower in fear.

If you're in close quarters with a dog that's sizing you up, maintain a tall, confident posture and do not look the dog in the eyes or show your teeth as the canine may see this as threatening behavior. Never reach out or attempt to strike a dog that hasn't attacked—you may still be exacerbating the situation and causing a dog to attack that may have just been snarling to show their dominance.

In the event of a dog bite, protect your face and neck and grab anything you can to shove into the dog's mouth, from a water bottle to a shoe, while you're yelling for help. If necessary, shoving your arm farther to the back of a dog's mouth may cause them to be unable to bite more forcefully and even cause them to release their grip. If you must try this technique, attempt to wrestle your weight on top of the dog to pin it while its mouth is occupied with your arm. During an attack, your goal is always to get away and end the danger; use every chance to free yourself from the situation while calling for help.

Some folks carry dog repellent or pepper spray, or even a squirt gun to spray water in a dog's face, but I have one tried-and-true method for halting a dog in its tracks, and literally saw the most quizzical look pass across that pooch's face as I ran right on by: Bark. Loudly. Think of the loudest you've ever yelled at anyone and multiply that by 11. A loud, deep guttural WOOF! can be more than enough to stop an advancing dog immediately.

During Ragnar Relay in 2009, I was running in a rough area of Arizona during a time when some of the local Indian reservations were having huge problems with packs of wild dogs when I literally found myself two lanes of traffic away from a small pack of wild, aggressive dogs heading my way. I was busy running, so I must've looked like the perfect prey to this large German Shepherd and Doberman; they were attempting to dart between cars to get at me. With no buildings or structures to my left and right, once there was a break in traffic I had no choice but to stand my ground. Luckily, I had read an article sometime earlier about standing up tall (I'm 5'8" and 150 pounds—combined, these dogs were much larger than me!) and barking out a "stop" command as loudly as possible. Well, at no point in my life have I ever made a noise like this; my WOOF! caused both dogs to stop their agitated darting back and forth, raise both ears, and—I kid you not—look at me with amazement before completely, utterly losing interest in chasing me. That was it: one man-bark and it was all over, threat averted. I hope you never have to try it, but if you need to just make it loud and confident, let those dogs know you're in charge.

Remember, avoiding conflict and calmly walking away is the absolute best option. Caesar Milan even gets bit from time to time, and if "The Dog Whisperer" can't always predict a pooch's behavior, neither can you.

Running Alone

First off, never run alone in a dark or unfamiliar place if at all possible. Even if you know the area well, always try to run with a partner. Nearly everything on the list of "running safety" can be prevented or abated quickly if you have another individual along with you. If you have no alternative, then always do the following:

- Let friends or family know where you're going, what your route will be and how long you'll be gone. I may sound a bit paranoid here, but I can name three runners off the top of my head who'd be alive today if they had followed this advice.

- Always carry a cell phone. If it's a smartphone, you can turn on GPS updates to broadcast your whereabouts to your friends and family so they know exactly where you are.

- Carry a flashlight or wear a headlamp from dusk to dawn and wear bright clothing with reflective strips or a vest.

- Leave your tunes at home. Make sure you're aware of your surroundings, and that includes being able to hear animals or muggers (or worse) that may be on your route.

- Women and teenagers (hopefully there are no pre-teens running around in the dark) should carry a whistle. It's easier to wake or alert others with a whistle and a scream than just a scream. The whistle may also startle an attacker enough to give you some time to get away.

- Carry or wear your contact information in an easy-to-find place. There are multiple companies selling ID-style bracelets that can contain your information and emergency contact numbers, and it's a simple solution that can save your life!

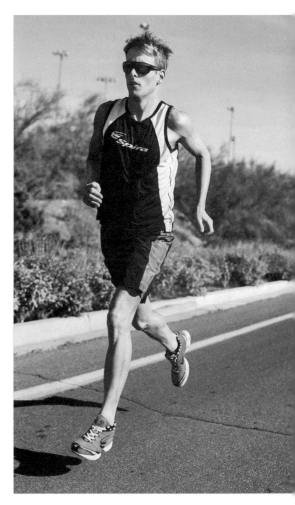

Most police agencies have programs to train the public how to use pepper spray properly in an emergency. If you're planning to run alone in the dark, it's a great idea to sign up and learn how to protect yourself. Run smart and stay safe. It's so much better to take the extra precautions and be safe rather than sorry.

Running with Your Head, Heart & Gut

Throughout any training run or race, there may be opportunities to speed up, obstacles that slow you down, and the highs and lows (see "The Highs & Lows of Endurance Running" on page 72) of exertion that will make you a little bit insane. (It's okay, we're all a little nuts.) During these different times, you'll need to run with other parts of your body that have nothing to do with the locomotion of your legs, feet and arms.

RUN WITH YOUR HEAD:

Focus on your form, tick off each mile while paying attention to your pace, breathing, etc. I've mentioned "run like a robot" a couple times, and running with your head is a lot like that. I use these times to take inventory on how my body feels during the run, how far I've run, how much is yet to come and calculate what I need to accomplish in term of pace or distance to meet my goals.

RUN WITH YOUR HEART:

Quite the opposite of running with your head, when you run with your heart you shut off the need to compute anything, you forget about your form (you don't sabotage your running form, you're just not obsessing over it) and just immerse yourself in the run. Yes, this is usually when your brain is flooded with endorphins and you're on a "runner's high," that euphoric feeling when dopamine takes control of your brain and everything just feels good.

RUN WITH YOUR GUT:

Sometimes a run can turn into an exercise in drudgery and you may find it difficult to continue; it happens to every runner, and sometimes it happens during every training run or race. Whether it's the suckiness of the first couple miles before you warm up, the downswing of the endorphin rollercoaster, or mental or physical fatigue,

there will be many opportunities for you to hone the necessary skill of running with your gut (better known as "embracing the suck") that will become necessary to keep you from quitting when times get tough. Strengthening your will to continue (aka "guts") is similar to building your endurance; it takes time, and the more you practice the better you'll become. When you get the desire to quit, having the mental fortitude to dig deep and keep pushing onward is essential to finishing your run. You may have heard the phrase, "Pain is temporary, quitting lasts forever," and while for the most part that's accurate, I'd like to make sure to qualify what the actual pain is. Pulled muscles, sprained ankles, gastric issues and especially any symptoms of cardiac problems (see page 28) means you should stop immediately. You should never keep pushing yourself if you're doing damage to your body. Period. In these situations, it's more important to "live to run another day." In situations where you're fatigued, sore or mentally disconnected and are thinking about quitting, it's time for a gut check. Think about how far you've come and how much work you've put in to get to this point. As long as you're not physically damaging yourself, you can usually finish the run based just on your guts.

How to Run

Running is a natural movement based on human physiology. Instinctually we'll run in times of crisis or fear (fight or flight response) or when chasing after objects or individuals (hunting, sports, the taxi that you just forgot your laptop in, etc.). I liken running form to the mechanics of nearly any other sport. Look at baseball, for example. Each player swings the bat differently, even after we're all taught the same basic skills in Little League. Adapting the swing to your own personal strength and style is the way you make it your own. Once you've developed that swing over time, it's extremely difficult—if not outright impossible—to change.

As I covered in the FAQs (page 19), you already know how to run—it's hardwired into your musculature as the most rapid form of personal locomotion. That being said, there are some tweaks to help you optimize your running output and some adaptations to your form that can help you run longer and healthier and even enjoy it a little bit more.

Note: "Proper running form" is different for every individual. Unlike the functional cross-training exercises, there's no one-size-fits-all description to follow. Read the tips and understand how they can potentially be of benefit, and then test them in training to verify the results.

Running Posture

A common phrase used in describing running posture that can be used as a mnemonic to remind yourself to keep good upper body form is "run tall." In order to be tall, you need to extend your torso, head and shoulders, not hunch over. Keep your chin up and your eyes looking

ahead whether you're on the road, trail or treadmill, scanning the area in front of you. This helps to keep your shoulders back as well—don't round them and hunch forward as this can limit proper arm swing, cause tension in your upper back and neck, and even inhibit full inflation of your lungs while breathing. Your back should be "straight," but that's a relative term since we all have our own comfortable position as it pertains to our posture. By bringing your shoulders and head back as if you were posing for a picture and reducing any bend at your waist to keep it as slight as possible, you'll experience the static version of "running tall." Now test it in your training!

With your back, head and shoulders straight, make sure to do the same thing with your hips by keeping your pelvis pointed straight ahead. After all, that's the direction you're running! To keep your hips in a relatively neutral position to allow proper range of motion for your legs, don't tilt too far forward or backward.

Tip: During sprints you'll bend slightly at the waist and lean forward, but you should limit this during jogging and normal running.

Your arms are partially responsible for the cadence your legs keep, but excess arm motion can tire you out, slow you down and even overly fatigue your core. Luckily, slightly modifying arm position is not nearly as difficult as changing the ingrained habits your legs have learned over the years. To keep from tiring out your core, focus on keeping both arms on the lateral sides of your body and not bringing your hands too far in front your body. After

TIP: In order to run and jog efficiently, you should be relatively relaxed from head to toe, but not "sloppy." When warming up or during periods when you're fatigued, you're most apt to lose your form and flail your arms and legs and essentially put your body in a poor running posture. Resist the urge to run like a toddler throwing a tantrum as it will only waste more of your precious energy and sap your muscle strength, perpetuate improper form and make you look like a three-year-old who wants to go get some ice cream (no matter how much you may desire some ice cream yourself at that exact moment).

all, you want your arms to swing freely and provide some of the motion that drives your legs forward, not excessively twist your torso with each swing. Your elbows should be bent about 90 degrees and kept close to—but not rubbing on—the sides of your torso. The more you flare your arms, hands or elbows while running, the more of your precious energy you'll waste, and the more you'll tire out muscles that don't need to be working that hard to keep you going efficiently. Squeezing your hands into tight fists will also waste energy and potentially cramp up your forearms, which in turn can sabotage your form. Keep your hands semi-relaxed with your fingertips touching your palms, wrists slightly relaxed but not flopping around.

Your legs and feet are usually the most natural part of running, and you already know how to use them to get from point A to point B as quickly as possible. Keep your stride short in front of your body and long behind you. Optimally, each foot should strike the ground with your heel, mid- or forefoot (we'll cover this later) directly underneath your body and push off from your forefoot to drive your body forward with each stride. By extending your leg too far out in front of your body and landing

> **TIP:** To reduce extra arm motion that can sap energy, I'll often try to mimic running like a robot and syncopate my arm and leg motion, keeping my shoulders loose and using the minimal amount of swing necessary to help keep my legs in motion.

> **TIP:** A good way to remember to keep your strides shorter and increase your turnover (number of strides per minute) is to make each step light and quick. One method is to listen to the sound your foot makes when it hits the ground and try to soften the impact and make it quieter. I'll often tell athletes I'm coaching or training to "run quietly" to help remind them to keep short, springy steps.

on the ground before it's underneath your body's mass, you're putting more stress on your entire body (specifically your knees, hips, lower back and even shins) than necessary.

Speaking of "springy" steps, a common waste of energy is bouncing too much with each step. The goal of running is to move forward as far or as quickly as possible, not upward. Since both feet will be off the ground a bit during each stride, there needs to be some upward lift. However, by limiting your entire body's lift for nearly 2000 steps per mile, you'll have more prolonged endurance during longer runs. Startling Fact: If you bounce just one extra inch with each stride over the course of a marathon, that additional upward motion alone would be close to climbing the Empire State Building three times!

Says Tricia Schafer, co-race director of the Night Run™, "It's so easy to take photos and videos of running stride these days with smartphones or even a head-mounted action cam. Work with a training partner and take turns videotaping or photographing each other on a track to examine race form. A power tip is to do it at the beginning when your muscles are fresh and running posture is proper, and then again at the end of your run when you've fatigued and have started to lose your form. Some of the most informative photos from races are the ones later on or at the end of the race, when my foot strike and form isn't quite as pretty as I'd like!"

Where the Rubber Meets the Road: Your Foot Strike

Even with optimal running form, each time your foot lands on the ground, the impact sends shockwaves through your body, originating from that foot through the bones, muscles, joints and tendons and eventually rattling around in your brain. Limiting the impact with each step should be a primary concern for each individual planning to run farther or faster.

A lot has been written about "proper" foot strike over the years, more recently with the advent of minimalist shoes and the revival of barefoot running due to the extreme popularity of Christopher McDougall's book *Born to Run*, in which he introduces the Tarahumara Indians in Mexico's inhospitable Copper Canyons as quite possibly the most adept distance runners on the planet.

Full disclosure: Let me go on record that I'm a fan of *Born to Run* and the real-life individuals who are portrayed in the book. Scott Jurek is an amazing person and one of the most accomplished ultra runners in the world; the late Micah "Caballo Blanco" True was a kind-hearted soul and running legend who was taken too soon; and Christopher McDougall himself is a well-liked and respected runner who occasionally makes it out to Arizona and runs in some of the same circles I do. *Born to Run* ignited a firestorm in the running community—and among shoe manufacturers. An entire new generation of runners has been inspired to run with and without shoes and over the past few years all the big shoe companies have gotten on board producing "minimalist" shoes. It's absolutely amazing what one book has done for the future of running!

How and where your foot makes initial contact with the ground on each stride is vitally important in how far or fast you run and how that impact affects the rest of your body. As I've mentioned numerous times already, everyone's running style is different and your physiology and adaptation of your gait over the years plays a huge part in how you develop a consistent foot strike. It should also be stated that as a runner becomes more fatigued, his or her foot strike will vary depending on tightness of muscles, fascia and tendons. Even the most ardent forefoot or midfoot runners can be caught in photographs striking their heels near the end of a race. In turn, even the heaviest of heel strikers will prance on the balls of their feet when encountering a steep, rocky or technical section of trail. It's important to be a well-rounded runner and train in various conditions so that you're prepared to run with different foot strikes on varying terrain.

Instead of sparking a debate whether one foot strike is better than another or any particular shoe technology is better than another, here are some observations on the different regions of the foot and how landing on them may affect your running style.

- **LANDING ON THE BALLS OF YOUR FEET:** You should only be doing this in drills or sprints (such as those located in "Functional Cross-Training Exercises" on page 124), not running any distance longer than a hundred yards or so. Landing first on the balls of your feet allows you to use your Achilles tendons and calves to absorb the impact and then fire the calves and contract, pulling on the Achilles tendon to forcefully drive the foot back off the ground. In some instances, the heel may not even touch the ground, keeping your calves under tension throughout the entire movement. Best used in bounds, skips and short sprints, landing on your forefoot is for fast movements over a limited distance.

- **LANDING ON YOUR MIDFOOT:** Conventional wisdom pegs midfoot landing as being the most efficient way to strike the ground to limit injury. It's not as extreme as the forefoot landing in using primarily the calf as the sole source of support and cushioning, and offers the most musculoskeletal balance as your foot is impacting the ground directly under your body, with the center of your foot touching the ground directly in line with your ankle and lower leg. A slightly bent knee and a very small bend at the hips cushion the impact stride to stride. Here's the rub, though: A midfoot strike requires your entire foot to land on the ground simultaneously. So, in essence, a midfoot strike is really a stable total foot strike. It'll take a little practice to develop a smooth transition from midfoot landing to forefoot push-off when you're first getting used to this method without slapping your whole foot down; the timing is to just clear or brush your heel on the ground, then land with your weight on your midfoot and then transition to your forefoot—all within a second or so!

- **LANDING ON YOUR HEEL:** Nearly all of us are heel strikers since our heel hits first when we walk. The only sure way to rid yourself of heel striking is trying to jog barefoot on pavement—the pain of landing on your heel with all your weight will provide the immediate feedback you need to transition to your midfoot or forefoot to absorb as much of that shock as possible. Try it for yourself; it's a jarring experience. Running in barefoot or minimalist shoes will have a similar effect—the lack of cushioning will force you to land in a more biomechanically efficient method to reduce the harshness of every landing. Now here's where I'll differ from the minimalists' marketing messages and blog posts: Heel-striking is not necessarily bad at all. "Barefoot-style" runners are known to extol the evils of running in thick, cushioned shoes that absorb heel impact and occasionally point to shoe companies as the devil incarnate, but, as I mentioned earlier, even the most efficient midfoot runners in the most high-tech minimalistic shoes will strike their heels from time to time as conditions and terrain change and fatigue sets in.

I strongly recommend everyone spend some time exercising barefoot on the grass. I'll sprint, bound and jog barefoot on grass every chance I get as it keeps my feet and calves strong and there's nothing quite as liberating as feeling the soft grass beneath my toes.

Stride Length, Running Gait & Foot Turnover

"Overstriding" is a term used to describe hitting the ground too far in front of your body. This impact causes your knee, hip and ankle to be in a weaker, less stable position than when landing below your body and actually causes a slight braking motion that slows you down when your heel hits the ground. An efficient stride or runner's gait consists of a small knee bend and lift to the front (but not exaggerated like a sprinter's leg raises), and landing with your foot directly below your body while transitioning your weight to the

forefoot and then pushing off and raising your leg with bent knee to bring your heel toward your buttocks. Without getting into the unnecessary minutiae of examining every nanosecond of each swing and stance phase, that's it. If you're hungry for every tiny little detail but aren't a professional athlete working to shave that last second off your 5K time, you may be over-thinking it!

Your foot turnover is just a fancy term for how often your feet hit the ground in a minute. Want a neat stat? Optimal turnover is often listed at 180, meaning each foot strikes the ground 90 times in one minute. Of course, your results may (and will) vary, but by taking short, quick strides and landing with your foot below your body, you can optimize your turnover. See "Functional Cross-Training Exercises" starting on page 124 for some drills designed to increase leg strength, speed and foot turnover.

This concludes an extremely low-tech lesson in Running 101. Hopefully you picked up some good tidbits to test out on your next few training runs to see what works best for you. Remember, don't try to change everything at once! If you've been running for one way your whole life, it'll take some time to make adjustments to your style so be patient. You'll also experience some soreness by changing drastically from a heel strike to midfoot, as your calves and Achilles tendons will be recruited into action to perform more shock-absorption duties in the landing phase.

How & Why You Should Build a Base

The phrase "building a base" or upping your "base mileage" quite simply refers to training. As with any other sport, you can't just hop in and immediately have the same strength, agility, coordination and endurance to compete at a high level as others who've trained and practiced. In running, "practicing" is actually just lacing up and running! While there are plenty of drills and exercises we'll cover in the workouts and programs, you can't improve as a runner without running—just like you can't improve as a soccer or basketball player without practicing your dribbling skills. You need to participate in sport-specific activities in order to be able to perform sport-specific activities.

Luckily in running, locomotion is the only real skill needed, and you don't need to spend years perfecting your form as you would jumpshots in basketball or learning to hit a knuckle curve in baseball. In order to be a runner, you need to run. The more you run, the faster, stronger and more aware of your body you'll be—in essence, you'll become a better runner.

By building a base, you not only develop the strength and endurance you need to run faster or longer, you also build up the muscles and connective tissue that allow you to keep running without injury. This process takes some time, and trying to do too much, too fast is a recipe for an injury that can sideline you and waste all the positive momentum you've built. By developing a consistent training program you can easily progress from a complete novice runner to an endurance athlete over time. How do I know? Because thousands of people do it every year—my clients have done it and so have I.

How do you build a base? The simple answer: You need to spend time running. The complicated answer includes:

- Walk/run intervals

- Long, slow distance (LSD)

- Speed sessions

- Tempo runs

- Pick-ups

- Hill repeats

- Cross-training

- Warm-up, cool-down and recovery runs

We'll cover those in "Interval Progression Training" starting on page 77, but it's easiest to say that during various times in your training you'll employ one, multiple or a mix of all the above running or cross-training workouts to build your base. Often, the term "base mileage" is only concerned with LSD and upping that weekly total for your long run by 10% from week to week. I disagree with that assertion, as all your mileage counts. From your slowest walk/jog when you're first starting out to 50-yard speed sessions, every mile you run has the ability to build up your base, and in excess they all have the power to knock you off your game with overtraining.

There's also no perfect number for what your base should be prior to your first or fastest 10K. I'll give some guidelines in the programs, but each individual reacts to training differently and it's much more important to develop long-term training habits that are conducive to training and fitness for the rest of your lifetime versus preparing for just one event. If you're looking for a cheat sheet on how to run one race and cross it off your bucket list, this may not be the book for you. My goal is to help you find a healthy balance with training that works with your lifestyle (or requires just some minimal changes to make it fit) and developing a consistent, progressive training program that will help you hit your goals this month, next month and years down the road. When I speak of "building a base," I'm referring to developing a healthy long relationship with running that will continue to grow for years to come.

Setting Goals

Hitting your goals is often extremely tricky, especially if you don't have any concrete ones. "Becoming a runner" or "finishing my first race" are great goals in their own right, but they're pretty subjective. If you go out for a jog every so often, you can probably tell your coworkers that you've become a runner, and dashing past a bunch of kids at a 1-mile fun run could clearly be considered finishing your first race, right?

Now, I'm not saying you should start off by setting some stringent, lofty goals like "break 40:00 for a 10K before January 1" or anything like that. Small goals that are relative to you and your lifestyle are usually the best way to start—but feel free to dream of lofty goals for a time a little ways off. First and foremost, you need to get on a successful running regimen in order to meet ANY goals. This starts with consistency. Here are a couple goals to give you a basic idea how to wrap your mind around goals that will help motivate you toward success.

BEGINNER GOAL: "I will run Monday, Wednesday and Friday for three weeks."

Simple and straightforward, this doesn't rely on any pace, distance, or exertion level. This goal is all about developing consistency to get you out the door thrice per week on specific days. Being specific about waypoints in your goals is as important as giving an address when trying to use a GPS; the more vague you are, the more second-guessing, frustration and desire to quit will take over.

Why it works: Setting specific days doesn't allow for procrastination—Monday means Monday. If you had a rough morning, sneak in a mile at lunch, after work, on a treadmill, before dinner or maybe a late-night jog before bed. When you give yourself a deadline, you're more apt to stick to it. Three times a week is extremely reasonable, and the every-other-day cadence has built-in rest days between sessions. The three-week duration is short enough that you can rationalize it as being simple enough to handle ("Heck, I can do anything for three weeks!") while being long enough to help you develop a routine. See "Why 7 Weeks?" on page 17.

How to fail: "I will run three days a week" allows you to put off that Monday run to Tuesday or Wednesday, then run twice on Friday…yeah, you see where this is going. You don't build a repeatable, consistent routine by being vague with your goals.

How to make it work: Write your running days on your calendar or input them into the reminders, tasks or alerts on your smartphone—whatever it takes to help you remember that you have an appointment with yourself that you're not going to break. I've found that putting my running gear by the end of the bed and setting my own alarm allows me to get up and out the door for a morning run with minimal interruption of my loving wife's glorious REM sleep.

"If you want to become a faster runner and hit your time goals, you need to come to the realization that if you want to race fast, you're going to have to train fast too. Specifically selected runs should include tempo runs, intervals or pick-ups at high intensity with recovery in between. Training your body to recognize speed feeds the mind and works your muscles, preparing you to replicate that effort on race day."
  —Dan Cadriel, elite amateur triathlete, sub-3:00 marathoner

If you plan on running at lunchtime, make sure you block off your online calendar by creating a repeating meeting for Monday, Wednesday and Friday. When coworkers are planning to sabotage everyone's lunch hour (seriously, who books a meeting at lunchtime?), they know in advance that you're already unavailable. Just make sure you stick to it. A simple tip for running at lunchtime is to leave before your fellow workers can entice you with an invite to the burger joint; you made your plans and you're going to stick to them. Speaking of making something, it always helps to pack a lunch for the days you'll be running since you're going to be cutting into your lunchtime and you don't want to waste your effort by grabbing fast food—and you won't stick to your new routine if you're missing lunch! Not only will the hunger pangs make the rest of the day miserable, you'll probably overeat when you get home. Pack something small like a sandwich and a yogurt; wash it down with a nice big glass of water. Save the sports drink for runs longer than 45 minutes, otherwise you're taking in more calories than you just ran off!

Tip: Running at lunchtime means you'll probably need to clean up before heading back to the office. If you're not using gym facilities with a shower, then baby wipes or sport wipes usually work great for all but the sweatiest of individuals on the hottest of days. Plan ahead: Pack some deodorant, wipes and baby powder along with a change of socks and underwear and you should be able to tidy up in the restroom stall pretty effectively in only a few minutes.

> "Running fast is all about stringing together quality daily runs over an extended period of time. The longer you work to maintain that consistency, the faster you'll get."
> —Lewis Elliot, professional triathlete, U.S. National Cycling champion

ADVANCED GOAL: "I want to set a new PR at X race on X date."

A very specific and focused goal, setting a new PR doesn't happen without a lot of hard work and dedication as you progress to your goal. More importantly, it doesn't happen without setting a sustainable, consistent routine like you did in the Beginner Goal, right? Most runners who've been in the sport continue to strive for farther distances or faster times (to a point) and most likely have subjective times they'd like to beat that are based solely on distances or what others may be able to attain.

Why it works: It's important to use the term "PR" versus an exact time, as it gives some additional wiggle room for you to consider a race a success by lowering your best time, while still not hitting some arbitrary time goal. For example, breaking 20:00 in a 5K is a very noble goal, but if your PR is currently 21:20, you have a higher potential for success giving yourself that additional 1:21 cushion. You're always racing against the clock in timed events, and fighting for that last second can be extremely frustrating if the stars don't align. On the flip side, by using a somewhat relative phrase of "setting a new PR," you may find yourself more relaxed and run even better than you expected. I chopped nearly 20:00 off my marathon PR by focusing less on my splits and more on how I was feeling during the run.

How to fail: Putting too much pressure on yourself to nail every training run and make everything perfect on race day. You can't control everything, and unless you're a professional it's nearly impossible to shut off the rest of your life and focus on running. Heck, even the professional athletes I work with can never truly figure it out 100% of the time. Stuff happens— you're going to miss workouts, have bad races and have to deal with suboptimal conditions in training and even at the big event. Every serious runner that I know has had more than their fair share of disappointments and it has been their resiliency to come back after a let-down to chase their PRs at a future event that makes them successful. Time and time again, the race you're planning to be perfect in every way rarely is; often, it's the next event when all your ducks are in a row and you do something special.

How to make it work: It all starts with the realization that with proper training, rest and execution on race day, the average

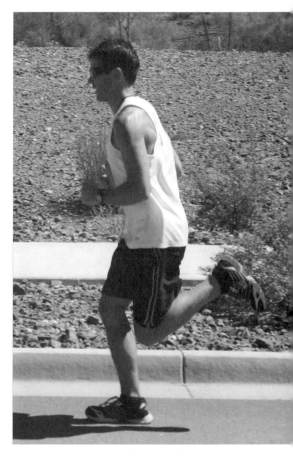

runner can continue to improve their best time. Because your PRs are relative to the only person who truly matters in your running career (you!), you can focus on making strides (pun intended) to progressively get stronger, smarter, healthier and faster.

Finding Your Motivation

Running really isn't that hard—you find some time to get out and run. Whether it's barefoot in the park with your kids, on a hilly mountain trail, treadmill or the pavement each morning, running is running. For some people, keeping motivated to stick with a running program can be extremely difficult.

The programs in this book are designed to give you a framework to develop good running habits and ward off some of the monotony of traditional boring routines, but they can't do all the work for you. You'll need to get off the couch and tackle your workouts in order to continue to make progress. Here are some ways to find your motivation and keep you focused on your training.

Running Buddies: They make it much easier to keep your routines on track. Knowing you have others who are alternately counting on and supporting you is an extremely good thing. In order to make a group dynamic work, you both need to take turns being the motivator. We all have our off-days where it's hard to get psyched up for a workout; that buddy nagging you over the phone to hurry up and get dressed to meet him for a run can be exactly what you need to get you fired up! Being accountable to other members of a group is a powerful motivator, especially if you don't want to get left behind.

Try it: Check out your local running store in person or online to find a wealth of group runs, running or triathlon clubs, local track workouts or even beginner programs for newbie runners. Know a coworker who runs? Ask them to tag along for a lunchtime jog and you may build a totally new connection! The best way to find others to run with is to be open and friendly and chat with others in your neighborhood or around the office who are into running. There's no shortage of online sites and social networks/communities for running junkies; from group runs and get-togethers to individuals sharing routes or even their workouts for the day, you can almost definitely locate other runners in your area. I've even seen running groups in Nome, Alaska.

How about starting your own running group? It's not as hard as it seems, and the easiest way to do it is to go out and run on a regular basis. Coworkers, friends and neighbors will see your positive example and eventually get around to asking to join you. Trust me, you're a motivator of others and you don't even know it yet!

Written Programs: Following a written program takes so much guesswork out of deciding when and how to exercise, and it also keeps you accountable for specific training times or distances. After all, the sheet says to run for three miles today, so I have to, right? Luckily, I've developed a few programs for you to use right here in this book, along with a log where you can keep track of your workouts and even keep notes about your perceived effort, nutrition and any other pieces of information you may find interesting: "Tuesday: Cute guy walks Schnauzer on 43rd Ave. around 10 a.m." Did I mention running is a great way to meet people who have the same interests as you? I shared Tricia and Johnny's story on page 36, but even if you're not single you can make some great friends and even clients!

As a writer and trainer, I create a lot of different fitness or nutritional regimens for my friends and clients as well as to hit my own goals. Without question, I'll follow a written program much more successfully than a list in my head—even if I wrote it myself! When an exercise is printed in black and white, there's no ambiguity about it; do these exercises for this many reps and then move on. When it's in your head, you can talk yourself into modifying every little piece of the workout based on how you feel. Once you make the smallest change to the reps or duration, you're more likely to derail the entire session by quitting early when "that's good enough" or even going harder and longer than you should and risk overtraining or injury. During exertion, your mental focus changes—keeping the workout in your head becomes more difficult and inaccurate as you progress through a training session, so bring a list or a log along to keep you on track and check off each exercise or drill as you finish. If you don't feel like lugging around a book, you can jot a small (but descriptive) list or use a smartphone to track your progress. We created an app that you can use with most mobile devices to help you out too. Check out www.7weekstofitness.com and click "apps" to learn more.

Technology: Technology can benefit your running by providing some motivation or even a release from some of the monotony of workouts. Hopefully I provided enough excitement in the programs in this book that you won't feel too bored, but realistically you may need to take your mind off your exercise from time to time. I covered running with music earlier, and even if the gym you're at doesn't have a TV, with a smartphone or tablet you can catch up on sports or movies on a treadmill. One of my running partners Michael Bennett will listen to audio books during ultramarathons and will usually finish a couple entire novels during a 24-hour event and actually learn something. Now that's multitasking!

Tip: When watching a video on a treadmill, don't be "that guy" laughing out loud to a movie or get too wrapped up in the action that you step off the belt and get flung off the machine. It happens all the time, but let's try to avoid that, okay?

Rewards: Treat yourself to a shopping trip when you hit goals or waypoints along the way. This will keep you focused on sticking to your routine when you want to pick up some new shoes, exercise clothes or even a new fitness gizmo. By keeping it focused on giving yourself a gift that will help you keep training, you compound the benefit! You worked so hard to deserve those fancy, expensive running shoes, now you need to use them! Whether you're a guy or a gal, showing off your new physique in well-fitting and comfortable clothes is a win-win; the confidence you get by looking good will help propel you to keep motivated in your workouts.

Tip: Don't use food or sweets as a little gift for a good workout; you may end up taking in more calories than you just burned off! Rather, choose items that will support your endeavor—purchase a few new tracks to add to your music library, replace your worn-out socks or test out some new anti-chafe products.

The Ass-ivation Scale

Let's face it—some days we all feel like we need a good reason just to get out of bed in the morning. I have a great gig writing books and training some awesome folks, but there are plenty of times when I'd like to smash the alarm and bury my head under the covers. Running is the same way for most people—if you can think of any reason to skip a daily run, they probably will. I'll admit to missing my share of workouts, but it never seems to be worth it: when I skip one, I just ending up paying for it later with a subpar performance at a race or even feeling miserable because I feel like I've let myself down. Usually the penalty is worse and lasts longer than the workout would've anyway. My wife can always tell when I'm cranky and has even thrown me out of the house to go for a run and cheer-up—and it actually works!

Ninety-nine percent of the time, we feel like superheroes after a good run or workout. Our endorphins are all cranked and we feel absolutely bulletproof. If we could bottle that experience we'd be millionaires...but more importantly, if we just remind ourselves how great we'll feel when we're done with the training it makes it that much easier to get psyched up for it. The remaining 1% of the time we either forget our running shoes or something. It happens to all of us.

Often misattributed to Beethoven, Ignacy Paderewski mused, "If I miss one day of practice, I notice it. If I miss two days, the critics notice it. If I miss three days, the audience notices it." Fitness is similar yet not exactly the same as a world-renowned musician skipping out on hours of playing scales. We all miss workouts, that's a given; the goal is to find your motivation and make it to far more than you miss.

The bottom line with motivation is that you'll never get through any life change without it. You need to be motivated to change jobs, try a new restaurant, even brush your teeth. Some motivation is easier (and smellier) than others, but every modification to your course of action requires you have the incentive to give it a shot and the follow-through to stick with it.

Here I introduce what I like to refer to as my "ass-ivation" scale, progressive levels of motivation from getting active through developing athletic performance:

Get off your ass-ivation: This is the most common motivation with individuals as they become more sedentary. It'll usually involve an epiphany after finishing off a bag of chips on the couch or just not fitting into your favorite jeans anymore. No matter what Mick Jagger sang back in 1964, time is not on our side, and every day, month or year you spend inactive you're gaining weight, losing athletic ability, stamina and cardiovascular fitness, and letting your body go to pot.

Lose my ass-ivation: This is weight loss and toning, usually for a life event like a wedding, beach vacation, class reunion or newfound single status that forces you to look somewhat presentable to others. Starting a running regimen is really popular with this group because they're usually looking for immediate results.

Kick some ass-ivation: This involves athletic improvement or sport-specific training for an upcoming season or events. Speed, core strength, endurance and flexibility are a common focus for most sports that involve getting from point A to point B as rapidly as possible, especially running!

Now, these top-three "ass-ivation" goals aren't mutually exclusive. You can lose weight, get healthy, improve your athletic ability and develop a fantastic physique all at the same time. Heck, that's what the programs in this book (and a few of my other fitness books as well) were created for! Using the "Settting Goals" section (page 64), you can begin your preparation and kick your plan into gear by using the Level 1 or Level 2 programs you'll find starting on page 101.

The Highs & Lows of Endurance Running

Much has been said about "hitting the wall" in a marathon at or around the 20-mile mark, and there may be some truth to it as a physical limitation for some, but for the most part it's entirely mental. In any endurance event, your mind will be your best friend and your worst enemy—all in the span of a few minutes. There'll be amazing highs where your heart will flow with boundless love for the spectators or an aid station worker handing you a cup

of water, followed immediately by feelings of self-loathing and outright anger toward other competitors, the course or that floppy shoelace that's driving you insane.

The worst part? You'll have no idea when it'll happen. Even during the best race of your life, as you push your body, your mind will fluctuate between light and dark. These highs and lows are relatively universal in endurance racing, so you're not going nuts if you alternate between Dr. Jekyll and Mr. Hyde out on the course.

The best way to deal with these waves is to enjoy the highs and be careful not to push yourself too hard while you're feeling like a superhero. When the lows come, you need to breathe deeply, relax and remind your neurons who's in charge. If the thought of quitting pops into your head, just remember how far you've come and how bummed you'll be later if you bow out now.

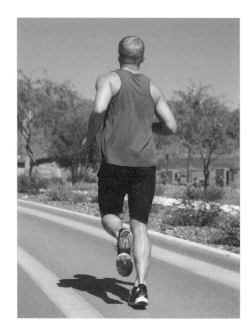

Rest: The Secret Weapon

Rest is not being lazy. When do your muscles grow? During your run, or afterward? It's an easy question to answer: during the downtime between runs. Did you realize that when you stress your muscles with exercise, you're actually tearing them? Don't worry—it's actually a good thing and not nearly as bad as it sounds. These microtears caused by strenuous or continual use of the muscles are an important step in the process of making your muscles grow stronger as they heal. Muscles repair themselves most when you're sleeping and continue during your off-days from training. Don't be tempted to "run a little" on those days—give your body time to heal. Since you're going to be adapting to a new routine and building up the distance and intensity of your workouts progressively, take advantage of all the time off allotted.

As I covered in "Overtraining" on page 29, your body needs to heal between workout sessions, otherwise you're risking injury and the litany of issues associated with overtraining. The worst part? All the "extra" training you're doing is only making you slower and delaying your body's ability to heal itself.

Here are some of the same tips used by professional athletes to maximize their recovery and boost performance:

Get at least 8 hours of sleep every night. That includes weekends too! Your circadian rhythms are easily knocked off-balance by late-night partying (or book writing).

Minimize any exercise or activity within one hour of bed. By the time you hop into the sack, your heart rate should be at a resting level.

Turn off your electronic devices. Living rooms are for TVs, bedrooms are (mostly) for sleep. Leave your mobile device, laptop or tablet in the other room; lit-up screens have been shown to disrupt early sleep patterns and keep you from falling asleep quickly. Falling asleep with the TV on generally means you'll stay up far later than you intended and only nod off when the infomercials start airing, right?

Turn off your brain too. Your bedroom should be a peaceful, relaxing sanctuary where you sleep and escape from all your stresses. Worrying does not promote a restful state, and you most likely won't fix your issues while you're in bed. Maximize your mattress time effectively by getting quality sleep.

Set the scene for rest. Keep your room dark with heavy curtains to block as much light as possible and use a fan or noise machine to provide a soothing sound to lull you to sleep.

Fuel your body to build muscle during sleepy-time. Protein provides the critical amino acids that serve as building blocks for the formation of new muscle. Casein and whey are the two non-soy protein powders you'll find at nearly any grocery or health-food store. While whey is metabolized quickly and should be taken immediately after a workout, casein protein is metabolized slowly and perfect for keeping your body anabolic while you're asleep.

Find the right bed for you. Lastly, every elite athlete I know loves their bed, or keeps searching for one until they do. Thirty-three percent of your life is spent sleeping—searching out the right bed is a very sound investment, and it doesn't necessarily need to be the most expensive, high-tech one either. If you're still lethargic in the morning or wake up with aches and pains, you haven't nailed the optimal one yet. While I can't say which bed is right for you, I can implore you to swap out a mattress that's robbing you of quality recovery time for one that allows you to get deep, restful sleep. During the writing of this book I replaced a five-year-old expensive pillow-toppy-cloud-softish dreambed for a very cheap firm mattress and have been rewarded with faster times falling asleep each night and waking up earlier, fresher and with more vigor to start my day.

Preparing for the Programs

Before we jump right into the programs, I'd like to cover some of the terms you'll be seeing throughout the workouts. In the three different levels, there will be lots of intervals at varying intensities, and the intensity, speed and distance will increase as you get farther along into the workouts. In other words, you'll be on the cutting edge of running training. With Interval Progression Training, each workout will build on the previous one in order to make you a stronger, faster athlete.

Your intensity is a big part of the workouts and, along with pace, is controlled solely by you. Your pace and intensity are relative to your fitness level and goals, so it's all up to you!

Exertion Scale

Here are the quick definitions of perceived exertion based on ability to hold a conversation, and obviously these are relative to the fitness and conditioning of each individual and will change as you become fitter. My running partners usually wish I'd shut the heck up—somehow I manage to run my mouth through almost any condition!

Easy: You should be able to carry on a conversation and breathe relatively normally. An easy pace is good for warm-up, cool-down, recovery the day or two after a hard-run race, or when running long distances. Easy runs or jogs are roughly 40–65% of your maximal effort.

Moderate: Your breathing should be faster than normal due to your elevated heart rate and exertion. While you can't carry on a full conversation, you can speak in occasional sentences. Moderate, or tempo, runs help to build strength and endurance. Moderate runs are about 65–85% of your maximal effort.

Hard: This is all-out sprinting. You'll be breathing extremely hard and unable to speak more than a word or so at a time. Hard intervals are done for a short period of time to build speed and train fast-twitch muscle fibers to respond even when fatigued. Hard runs represent over 85% of your maximal effort.

Target Heart Rate & Zones

If you're a bit more attuned to data and happen to own a heart monitor (or like to do math), you can use the following Attainable Heart Rate equation to calculate your Target Heart Rate (THR). *Note:* This is not exact and can fluctuate by as much as 15 beats per minute (BPM); use this only as a guideline (note: 100% = maximal effort).

$$(220 - AGE) \times ZONE \% = THR$$

ZONE 1 (EASY):
40–65%—WARM-UP & COOL-DOWN/RECOVERY

ZONE 2 (MODERATE):
65%–85%—AEROBIC ENDURANCE

ZONE 3 (HARD):
85%—PEAK ZONE/ANAEROBIC THRESHOLD

For example, a 30-year-old male looking for Target Heart Rate (THR) at a 70% effort has a THR of 133 BPM:

$$(220 - 30) \times 70\% = 133$$

Whatever method you use, it's important to listen to your body and follow the recommendations. An easy effort shouldn't be at high intensity, and there's a good chance you shouldn't be chatting up your running partner during hill repeats!

Interval Progression Training

From day 1 of the Prep Program, I'll be starting you on a progressive program of interval training. That's right—none of that boring stuff that you may have expected like lacing up shoes and running. We're talking about high-tech, modern… what? Oh, intervals are running? Yeah, gotcha. Okay, you'll be running, but the goal will be slightly different than most other traditional programs. I'm providing you with a blended approach based on incrementing your weekly mileage while focusing on getting in as many shorter runs as possible at the desired intensity. The goal for all of the programs is quality over quantity to get stronger, fitter and, well, faster.

Prior to any training or racing, it's extremely important to warm up. Jogging easy is a great method to raise the heart rate, get your muscles warm and loosen up. Progress from a casual walk to a brisk walk, and then an easy jog for 5–10 minutes or up to a mile; then stop and perform a few dynamic stretches to loosen up your hips, quads, calves and lower back before you start training seriously. Voilà! You've already started your progression training, and that's just warming up!

Tip: Even when performing the cross-training workouts on days where you're not running, a walk/jog/stretch progression will get you ready for your training.

Here's an overview of how you'll progress through the programs. You'll build

your speed, strength and endurance while you also focus on specific drills that will give you the physical and mental fortitude to continue to run stronger later in races and nail your PRs.

Walk/Brisk Walk: We all have to start somewhere, and I'm sure you heard the phrase "you need to learn to walk before you can run." Walking will help you build your endurance while adding a healthy, active routine to your life. Not only that, walking at the right time (see Prep Program on page 88) will help you lose weight and prepare your body for running.

Walk/Jog: Whether you're a newbie just getting off the couch, a jogger returning from an injury or an elite runner, walk/jog intervals are part of your warm-ups or workouts. Sometimes to get fast you need to start out slow (this is one of those times!). Both play a big part in running, and these intervals are great training for any distance, any level or any athlete. I've personally used run/walk intervals in marathons and ultramarathons as well as during an Ironman triathlon with great results—they work! Get the mind-set out of your head that walking's bad—that's nonsense. Running with bad form is bad! Many trainers and coaches—including me—will recommend walking through water stations in order to catch your breath, hydrate and recover a bit during races. I like to call little walk breaks "adaptive recovery" where you're continuing to move forward while building your energy back up. A little break can go a long way to helping you continue a long run or race and it's important for you to embrace run/walk intervals during training as well.

Jog: The goal of the Prep Program is to build up your jogging consistency and distance. This starts as an easy effort and progresses to a moderate exertion over longer distances, especially as you start to build consistent speed. Prior to dialing in any consistent speed bumps, I'll teach you a little something about developing a pace. See "What Shelby Taught Me about Pacing" on page 80.

Tempo: Tempo runs are an extremely effective method for developing speed and endurance, and they're the cornerstone of the Prep, Level 1 and Level 2 programs. A "tempo" pace is relative to each individual, so until you establish a "race pace," I'll define it as a moderately hard effort that you can maintain for the prescribed amount of time. In jog/run tempo runs, you'll be performing intervals at tempo followed by rest and recovery jogs.

Tempo/Speed: Building on the jog/tempo runs, the tempo/speed runs are moderately hard runs for a period of time followed by a faster run for a short duration. These speed "pick-ups" are designed to build speed by pushing the pace even when you're fatigued. These drills are the secret to finishing strong and even locating "another gear" or finding speed you never knew you had. Commonly known as the "Holy *bleep* Moment," you'll never forget the first time you experience the turbo boost of hitting that next gear.

Speed/Power: Flat speed is fine and dandy, but how many road courses are completely flat? You'll need to develop your leg strength with intense, short power workouts over elevated terrain. Yes, these are the sometimes-dreaded "hill repeats"! Quick yet effective, these drills are hard exertion for as little as 20 seconds followed by a recovery walk or jog before repeating. Speed/power drills will also help to make you a stronger and more durable runner. The heavy workload put on your legs to propel you up the hills at a high rate of speed are notorious for being a secret weapon for most elite athletes who engage in football, soccer, skiing, triathlon and many more.

Taper: See "Jog" above. This is the seven- to ten-day period before your race where you'll be slashing your mileage and speed, giving your body time to rest and recover while still putting in enough of an effort to stay loose and keep you from going nuts. (See "Taper" in the FAQs on page 26.)

Understanding Your Pace

"Your pace or mine?" Aside from sounding like a cheesy pick-up line, this is actually an important question to ask of your training partners or coach, or even a reminder to yourself when choosing a group to train or pace with at an event. Determining your pace is important for many reasons:

- Knowing your pace allows you to determine how long it will take to cover a given distance.

■ Knowing the time duration (based on your pace) of your run allows you to make hydration and supplemental nutrition decisions based on an accurate timetable as opposed to when you "feel like it" (see Pacing by "Feel" below).

Once you know your pace, you can use that knowledge to more accurately judge distances on an unmarked course, and most importantly you can explain to your significant other when you'll be home from a run or even calculate where and when they can see you on the course during a race.

However, there's a bit of a catch: Your pace is completely relative to you and it changes based on many, many variables such as distance, conditions, temperature, your mental and physical preparedness, and about 3000 other micro-variables[1] (from loose shoelaces to an extralong line at the port-o-potty). I like to use the term "relative pace" as a whole, and then specifics based on distance or conditions (examples: relative 5K pace, relative trail 10K pace, relative freezing-cold-5-miles-in-the-rain-spent-cursing-the-weatherman-and-dreaming-of-a-hot-chocolate pace). Since every race course is different, you'll have a specific pace in relation to different ones. Here are a couple of mine: The Night Run 8K pace, Thursday-night Road Runner Sports 5K pace, Runner's Den 10K Trail pace, Castle Craig "Tradition Run" 5K Up pace, and the 5K Down pace.

"But wait a minute, I was told I should be running at a 8:00 pace for a 10K and a 7:46 for a 5K blah blah blah blah blah…." Sure, races are timed—that's a given—and the calculation of the time spent from the start to finish line divided by the distance actually is your pace for that race, that time. (If you run the same course 15 more times, you'll most likely have 15 different results due to the micro-variables I mentioned earlier.) In order for any pace per mile to have any context in relation to your running ability, you need to put in the time and effort to develop knowledge of how fast you can run with a certain amount of exertion for a given period of time. (See "Exertion Scale" on page 76 or the quick reference table on page 80). It may sound like a cop-out, but you simply won't know what your pace is until you put in the work to develop it.

If you've never run any timed distance of 5K or more, it'll take a little time, patience and practice to develop your pace. Luckily, in the interim you can use the exertion scale to give you a rough idea of how hard you can run for a given distance. Of course, you'll need a little while to get "up to speed" (pun intended) and you should start off with the Prep Program on page 88.

PACING BY "FEEL"

During training and especially at events, you're thinking about way too many different things to accurately judge

---

1   Micro-variables: All the stuff you don't realize that could possibly screw up your run. These include loose shoelaces, blisters, swallowing a bug, losing a contact lens, dropping an energy gel, inclement weather or changing temperature, etc. Essentially, it's Murphy's Law for Runners.

whether you're in need of hydration, calories, caffeine (if you take it), electrolytes, etc. For the most part, when you go by "feel," you're much more apt to forget something or make a mistake. A popular adage is "If you feel thirsty, then you're already dehydrated," and while the truth of this is often debated, simply having a plan based on time can alleviate any questions and trying to do calculations on the fly while you're on the course. Once you know your pace and can approximate the time it takes to cover a distance, you can easily make a mental note (or write it on your forearm with a Sharpie, like I've done) when to eat an energy gel, how often to drink water, when to gulp some sports drink or take some electrolyte tablets, etc.

See "Exertion Scale" and "Target Heart Rates & Zones" on page 76 for descriptions, but here's a handy-dandy little chart:

Exertion	Zone	Max. Heart Rate %
Easy	1	40–65%
Moderate	2	65–85%
Hard	3	85%+

It may sound a little bit counter-intuitive, as "listening to your body" is extremely important, but you need to train and race for a while in order to completely understand what's saying to you. In the case of nutrition or hydration during a race, it may actually be telling you too late for you to take the necessary actions! This also holds true for approximating your pace without a watch or on-course timer. Unless you've really spent some time learning what your different paces are for different distances, you're more apt to vary too much from your desired speed and intensity and either run out of energy too soon or miss your goals.

WHAT SHELBY TAUGHT ME ABOUT PACING

The first lesson that any decent running coach will teach a student who's planning to run any distance should be: "Start slow to warm up, run within your ability for as long as you can, slow down to cool off." My running coach was a little bit more mysterious when she first sought to teach me about finding and maintaining my pace: "Woof."

Shelby is my white bull terrier (think Target dog or Spuds MacKenzie) and has been my running partner for the last several years. My joy and excitement to go for a run is only second to her exuberance when she bounds from the gate for our daily jaunt around the neighborhood or a quick tempo run to the park for some calisthenics (me, not her) and then back. One thing Shelby taught me very quickly, whether we were running over snowy sidewalks in Connecticut or mountainside trails in Arizona, was that she has no idea whatsoever how to pace herself. Literally none. Her two speeds are "all on" or "full stop." Her exertion is always at one of the extremes—either she's frenetic or exhausted—and this all happens within the span of a few miles. Here's the play by play:

"Always start a race a little slower than your target goal pace and speed up as you can. This is called 'negative splits,' where your pace decreases each mile. Going out too fast is suicide in racing."

—Lewis Elliot, professional triathlete, U.S. National Cycling champion

- Mile 1, pace 7:02/mile: Like a yo-yo on fire, she darts back and forth and pulls at the leash with all her might, her little bully legs propelling her 65-pound body like a rocket up the sidewalk while I struggle to hang on and keep up.

- Mile 2, pace 8:23/mile: Not counting the two or three times she comes to an abrupt halt to water the bushes, her pace has dropped by nearly a minute and a half per mile. No longer pulling at her leash, she has dropped into a reasonable jog that's enjoyable for us both.

- Mile 3, pace N/A. Occasionally being cajoled into motion toward home, Shelby has no real pace above a walk and occasionally will flop flat on the concrete and refuse to move for minutes at a time. No longer fun for both of us, it's now a battle of wills to persuade her to jog back home for some ice-cold water and a treat.

Now, how many of you can describe your running the same way? Are you exhausted after only a mile (or less) because you started way too fast? You're not alone, and it's extremely common for newbie runners to immediately jump on the gas and empty their tank too soon (at the O'Hartford 5K early in my running career, I posted a 5:35 for mile 1 only to follow it up with a 9:30 and the final 1.1 over 11:00). Even seasoned runners can find themselves caught up in the excitement of a start line and expend too much energy too early by jumping out too fast.

For your first race, you should only have the goals to finish and enjoy the experience—don't worry about beating anyone else or running your fastest. Because it's your first race, you'll automatically have a PR! Your first race should be a baseline for you to use to build your running career off of and hopefully continually improve on your time. Once your first race is in the books, you'll now have a real "race pace" that you can use to estimate your speed for all of your workouts.

If you're an experienced runner who's moving to a new distance or striving for a PR, you still need to heed the lesson of holding back and not going out too fast.

FINDING "ANOTHER GEAR"

In a 2010 study by Samuele Marcora and Walter Staiano of Wales's Bangor University, 10 male athletes were asked to pedal a stationary bike as hard as possible for 5 seconds, then rode the same bikes until they could no longer maintain a fixed rate of speed/power (90% of their individual VO2 max), considering this exhaustion. Immediately, they were asked to pedal as hard as possible for an additional 5 seconds. While they produced about 30% less than the initial 5-second test (when they were fresh and rested), the athletes produced 300% more output of speed/power than the 90% VO2 max test! In other words, even when the athletes were "exhausted," they still had enough energy and strength left to push their bodies 300% FASTER at the finish of the test. Apply this to the finish line at a hard training run or a race and you can see how athletes find the strength to overcome their fatigue and "kick it into another gear" during the home stretch.

Early on in running, I was lucky enough to tap into my "extra gear" and developed a pretty decent kick at the home stretch. I called it "smelling the finish line" and I could usually drop the hammer and run hard no matter how bad I felt. This served me well in triathlons when I was extremely spent but would summon the strength to finish strong. It wasn't until I rounded the final corner of the Night Run in 2011 that I learned I had one more gear. As we crested the top of the final hill and turned toward the finish line, another middle-aged runner pushed past me and headed into the home stretch. Not content to let him finish ahead of me, I kicked it up a notch and edged ahead as he began to falter. At the same time, I pulled ahead of Erik, a spry 12-year-old who thought I was challenging him in a sprint to the line. As his young legs started to churn, I figured "why not?" and pushed my legs into the red. To my amazement, they responded favorably. In a photo finish, the youngster and his three-decade youthful advantage edged me out, but I had learned a valuable lesson that I use with my clients today: Fatigue and even exhaustion are at least partially mental; you can nearly always push a little harder to finish. Try to remember this during the tempo pick-ups and fast finishes, as well as during the final stretch of any race!

Functional Cross-Training

Since the jogging craze's heyday in the early 1970s, running has been all about, well, running. Other sports were mostly based on that same train of thought: To be a better skier you skied every day possible, traveling the world to keep up with the snow. Baseball players spent more time fielding balls, shagging flies and getting every possible swing in the batting cage in between games. Golfers played golf. Period. Why would running be any different?

Fast-forward to the last couple decades, and you can see the enormous role cross-training has played in the physiques of athletes in every sport. Ballplayers got bigger and stronger and nowadays even golfers travel with personal trainers who put them through workouts nearly every day to ward off injuries by building strength and flexibility. Elite runners and triathletes have been benefitting from cross-training for years, and amateur running enthusiasts can reap the same benefits of stronger bodies producing faster times and longer endurance. Running is an extremely linear activity—when training by merely repeated running, muscles and ligaments are stressed in a limited manner, just to progress the runner forward while joints, muscles and connective tissue in the linear plane atrophy. Cross-training develops the entire body through multiplane movements, creating athletes that are stronger, more flexible and more resistant to injury. The end result is better all-around sports performance and longevity as an athlete.

Bodyweight strength training combined with running drills is an incredibly efficient way to build strength, endurance and speed as well as develop a lean, ripped physique. Let's be honest, though; none of us is perfect. Due to years of improper posture, sports injuries or even weak musculature, we all have imbalances that can affect proper form and even put us on the fast track to injury. In addition, jumping into a new exercise routine too quickly or doing the exercises with improper form can exacerbate any pre-existing injury. This is why we recommend starting out by performing each bodyweight exercise slowly and focusing on proper form.

Throughout the cross-training routines, you should expect to experience mild soreness and fatigue, especially when you're just getting started. The feeling of your muscles being "pumped" and the fatigue of an exhausting workout should be expected. These are positive feelings.

On the other hand, any sharp pain, muscle spasm or numbness is a warning sign that you need to stop and not push yourself any harder. Some small muscle groups may fatigue more quickly because they're often overlooked in other workouts. Your hips, glutes and core will be doing a tremendous amount of work and can easily tire out. If you're exhausted, take a rest. It's far better than using improper form and risking hurting yourself.

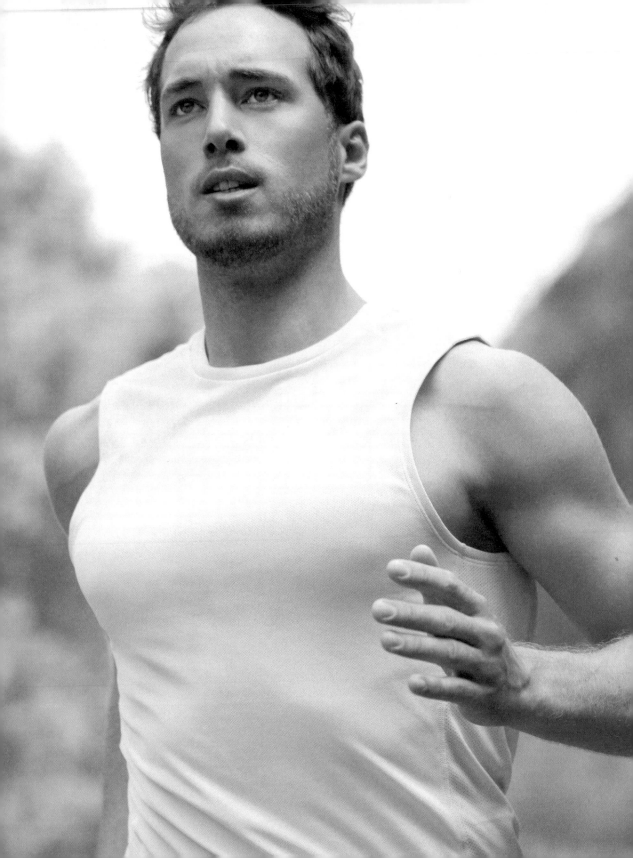

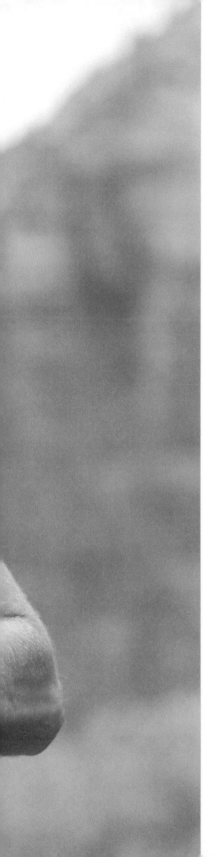

PART 3:
THE
PROGRAMS

About the Programs

"Listen to everyone, follow no one. Mostly, just get out there and run!"
—*DEAN KARNAZES*

While this book is focused specifically on the 10K distance, for the most part running is still running. The Prep, Level 1 and Level 2 programs can all quite easily be tailored to any distance from 5K through the 50K (31 miles). By modifying the training regimens a little bit, you can run your first or fastest 5K by following this program to the letter and totally stomp your goals—the extra mileage will only help you finish stronger and faster at the 3.1-mile distance.

If you're running any longer-distance races, progress through the Level 1 and Level 2 programs exactly as they are; the one modification is to extend the base mileage sections relative to your goal distance. For example, the marathon distance is roughly 42K, four times as far as a 10K. Multiply the longest weekly run by 4 to obtain the appropriate base mileage for your 26.2-mile training.

Prior to each workout, we'll spend at least five minutes warming up before even thinking about stretching out—you never want to stretch cold muscle fibers as it can cause damage and even muscle tears or trauma that could potentially sideline you for weeks! Repeat after me: Warm up first, stretch dynamically, work out, run or race, cool down a little bit and then stretch to start the recovery process. See "Warming Up" (page 135) and "Stretches" (page 138) for specific exercises.

Post-Run Cool-Down

The post-run cool-down should be a 3- to 5-minute jog where you descend from your training pace to a slow, controlled jog at about 50% intensity. You'll mitigate cramping, allow for enhanced blood flow to your muscles to lessen pain and fatigue, and help you bounce back for your next training faster by allowing your body to cool down while still in motion versus stopping and resting. During this period, you can begin to refuel with a drink of 4:1 ratio of carbs to protein (hint: chocolate milk works extremely well!) and then follow up with some specific stretches and a session with a foam roller to make you feel (almost) as good as new.

Reading the Charts

While the charts should be relatively self-explanatory, in order for you to get the most out of your workout, you should read through the exercise routine for that day and review proper form provided in the step-by-step instructions and photos in the "Functional Cross-Training Exercises" section beginning on page 124 and the running drills described before each program. The workouts for each day are listed vertically, and each are performed back to back with little to no rest in between unless a rest period is specifically prescribed.

Example: Level 1 Week 5 Monday (on page 108): You'll perform a 5-minute warm-up followed by a 1.5-mile easy run and 30-second walk/jog that's repeated once before a 5-minute cool down.

Note: Dark gray boxes indicate a workout that has two parts. Complete the required number of repeats in the light gray portion first, rest and then progress to the darker gray section. If you're time-constrained, you may split the workouts into morning and night sessions.

Prep Program

Welcome to the Prep Program. This is by far my favorite level to train individuals and introduce "newbies" to running. Why do I love it so much? Because you have the most to gain out of adopting a healthier fitness lifestyle through running, and you'll see the most gains in the shortest amount of time. Whether your goal is losing weight, getting off your butt, changing your daily routine, meeting new friends, getting into shape, reclaiming your body after having a baby or even preparing for your first race, the Prep Program is the crucial first step to a whole new you!

Who's the Prep Level good for?

- First-time runners (newbies)
- Those looking for a good introduction to cross-training
- Athletes coming back after an injury
- Individuals who've spent a long time away from training and need to get back into it
- New mothers looking to reclaim their bodies through fitness
- Anyone who wants to get fit, have fun and experience the cardiovascular benefits of walk/jog intervals and cross-training

Quite often, individuals turn to running in order to lose weight but are unable to run, walk or jog even a short distance before fatigue, muscle or joint soreness forces them to a halt. Aside from existing injuries, the two conditions related to these issues is that the individual is carrying extra weight or is in poor cardiovascular shape—and it's usually a combination of both. Don't worry; we'll tackle both those areas in the Prep Program simultaneously, enabling you to shed excess weight while training to become a runner. Even if you're not concerned with losing weight, read through the following section for important info about learning your BMI, BMR and how your body burns fat for fuel at specific times throughout the day.

Dropping Weight to Begin Running

Running can be a very effective way to lose weight quickly. I say "can be" because all too often people do it wrong and fail, no matter how far, fast or long they run. How can you run and not lose weight? Quite simply, they either overestimate the amount of calories they burn and overeat after they're done (covered on page 66) or they overestimate the number of calories they take in during and after their run. For instance, if you drink a full sports drink with around 300 calories and run less than one hour, you've actually taken in more calories than you've burned from that workout. Yes, this is amazingly common and knocks a lot of new runners off track. Also, running and cross-training make you hungry and if you refuel with less-than-optimal nutrition with excessively high carbs, bad fats (partially hydrogenated, some saturated) and even too much protein by eating huge portions, you'll actually gain weight. (See the cheat sheet on calories burned during running and calculating your basal metabolic rate on page 45.)

If you want to drop weight while you're running, the easiest and healthiest fast track to losing a healthy one to three pounds a week is by slightly modifying your physical activity and nutrition timetables. Essentially, exercising more and watching what—and when—you eat. Yes, that sounds like the same advice you've heard a million different times, but I try to make it as easy as possible by providing a guideline for when you should exercise, for how long and what meals to eat before and after in "Meal & Exercise Timing" (page 90).

First, it's necessary to assess your Body Mass Index, or BMI, in order to somewhat better understand what your plan of action should be to healthily start slimming down. (*Note:* BMI does not account for muscle mass so is relatively inaccurate in assessing muscular individuals, usually putting them incorrectly in the "obese" category.)

The BMI formula is a little complicated:

WEIGHT (IN POUNDS) / [HEIGHT (IN INCHES)]^2 X 703

Calculate BMI by dividing weight in pounds by height in inches squared and multiplying by a conversion factor of 703.

Example: Weight = 150 lbs, height = 65" (5'5")

Calculation: [150 ÷ (65)^2] x 703 = 24.96

(The U.S. Center for Disease Control provides an easy calculator online: www.cdc.gov/healthyweight/assessing/bmi.)

- If you're obese and sedentary (BMI higher than 25), you can drop between 1–3 pounds per week by adding 20 minutes of exercise (as little as walking or some simple calisthenics) to your regimen each day. Don't make any drastic changes to your nutrition at the same time. Take 2–3 weeks and focus on adding 20 minutes of exercise to your daily routine before adding in some of the meal timings noted below and nutritional suggestions.

- For those in the "normal" rating of BMI (18.5–24.9), you can see some positive results by adding 20 minutes of exercise if you're normally sedentary, and will see enhanced results by eating healthier food choices—more vegetables;

leaner, higher-protein meats, fewer processed carbohydrates; cutting down significantly on or removing snacks and fried foods from your diet. You can also limit your caloric intake as much as 500 calories below your BMR (see page 45).

- If you're below 18.5 on the BMI scale, you'll actually need to take in more calories while adding a running and cross-training regimen to your routine. Adding 200 to 500 calories in vegetables, lean meats, healthy fats (nuts, oils, avocados) and non-processed carbs will help you stay lean while also giving your body the fuel it needs to perform well under the new demands of a training routine.

Meal & Exercise Timing

The easiest program to lose weight quickly is to kick up your body's natural ability to burn fat and also extend your fat-burning "window" that your body enters into every night. When you sleep, your body has burned through its glycogen stores and overnight will burn a majority of fat as fuel to keep your systems running. As much as 60% of your fuel will come from fat— that's roughly equivalent to jogging at 45% intensity for most of the night, every night! Then again, that happens normally every night, so it's not like this is anything new for your body. In order to reap the benefits, you can extend that magic fat-torching window as long as possible. Here's a quick, general overview on how you can optimize that fat burn every day while starting the Prep Program and still going about your daily life.

NOTE: This meal and exercise timing is designed for maximizing weight loss before or during the Prep Program and is not intended to be used in conjunction with the Level 1 or Level 2 programs, which are much more intense and require a more balanced approach to nutrition, especially pre-workout carbohydrates. The nutritional program listed below has you "running on empty" in the morning to maximize fat burn, and is not conducive to high-intensity training.

6:00–7:00 a.m.: Start your morning off on a positive note with your daily "cardio" exercise from the chart. Need to grab a cup of coffee before you go? Go ahead, just make it black. Any carbs will immediately shut off your magic fat-burning state. Since you won't be performing high-intensity intervals or exercising for a long duration, you can get by without eating first. Take advantage of your body burning fat for fuel while you can!

8:00 a.m.: Eat a small breakfast that's high in protein and low in carbohydrates. Scrambled eggs, turkey bacon and a quarter avocado are tops on my list. Skip the toast, waffles and especially a muffin or scone—keeping your morning carbs low will avoid an insulin spike and the following crash that will leave you with a "case of the blahs" later in the day.

10:00 a.m.: Eat a half-cup of steel-cut oats topped with some fresh fruit—a little bit of protein and slow-burning carbs will help keep you satiated until lunchtime.

12:00 p.m.: Lunchtime? Not yet! For your noon workout, take a 5-minute walk to warm up, then perform your cross-training exercises from the chart for that day. Later on in the programs, I suggest jogging to a park to do your cross-training.

12:30 p.m.: Eat a sensible-portion lunch. Spinach salad, chicken breast and veggies are always a favorite; make sure to top with oil and vinegar—not any creamy (high-calorie) dressing!

3:00 p.m.: Carrot sticks, celery, quarter avocado in half a green pepper make a great, filling treat. Still hungry? Eat more carrots! If you need something "decadent," find a granola or snack bar with around 100 to 140 calories (not a 300+ calorie meal replacement bar) and a least 4g of protein to keep you satisfied until dinner.

6:00 p.m.: Eat a healthy dinner. For example, 4- to 6-ounce grilled, skinless chicken breast, 1 cup steamed broccoli, and 4-ounce sweet potato or quarter cup brown rice.

8:00 p.m.: End your day with an easy, relaxing evening workout—take a 20–30 minute walk to kick-start your fat burning before you head off to dreamland.

Bedtime: Then make sure you get at least eight hours of restful sleep.

The above regimen is really not that difficult once you make it part of your routine. Yes, the first week or so of any lifestyle modification can be a bit tough, but you're putting in the groundwork of a totally NEW YOU! Once you start to get used to eating healthy portions at specific times, you'll find it becomes much easier to stick with it. Here are a couple tips:

- If you want to stay on schedule, pack your lunches. Grill some chicken breast and put it in a sandwich bag separate from your veggies and spinach; combine them at lunch and they'll taste better than if they spent all morning combined in the office fridge.

- For veggies like carrots and celery, bring a huge bag and snack on them if you feel the urge. If you need some more flavor, choose hummus to dip in rather than a creamy dressing.

- That snack bar for 3:00 p.m.? Grab a black permanent marker and write "3:00 p.m." across it, and don't open it until it's time. Teach yourself that YOU'RE the one in control of your hunger, not the other way around.

- The secret to ending carb cravings (yes, they're completely for real—you're not going insane) is to stop eating bad carbs. Period. Seriously, each time you cut down on sneaking snack carbs (chips, breads, pastas, etc.) the easier it gets the following day. Unfortunately, as soon as you slip, you're back on the carb roller coaster all over again. Your body gets hooked on the fast-acting glucose as a quick high, but leaves you quickly in a low…and begs you to do it all over again. Break the cycle and reap the health and weight-loss benefits.

Note: Warm up for 5 minutes prior to intervals or cross-training; stretch after each workout (cardio intervals, cross-training). See pages 135–39 for Warm-Ups & Stretches. Use exertion scale on page 76 for Easy, Moderate and Hard effort.

Prep Week 1 Running & Cross-Training

Mon	Tue	Wed	Thu	Fri	Sat	Sun
20:00 morning walk	20:00 morning walk	20:00 morning walk	20:00 morning walk	20:00 morning walk	Morning: • 10:00 normal walk • 10:00 brisk walk *repeat*	30:00 morning walk
5 Hip Raises	20:00 evening walk	:20 Plank	20:00 evening walk	6 Mountain Climbers	20:00 evening walk	20:00 evening walk
5 Squats		4 Bird Dogs		5 Squats		
5 Supermans		4 Cobras		6 Supermans		
6 Flutter Kicks		8 Jumping Jacks		6 Hip Raises		
3 Push-Ups		8 Toe Touches		4 Push-Ups		
1:00 rest		1:00 rest		1:00 rest		
repeat		*repeat*		*repeat*		
20:00 evening walk		20:00 evening walk		20:00 evening walk		

Note: Warm up for 5 minutes prior to intervals or cross-training; stretch after each workout (cardio intervals, cross-training). See pages 135–39 for Warm-Ups & Stretches. Use exertion scale on page 76 for Easy, Moderate and Hard effort.

Prep Week 2 Running & Cross-Training

Mon	Tue	Wed	Thu	Fri	Sat	Sun
20:00 morning walk	20:00 morning walk	20:00 morning walk	20:00 morning walk	20:00 morning walk	Morning: • 10:00 normal walk • 10:00 brisk walk *repeat*	30:00 morning walk
:20 Plank	20:00 evening walk	6 Hip Raises	20:00 evening walk	6 Mountain Climbers	20:00 evening walk	20:00 evening walk
5 Bird Dogs		5 Squats		4 Lunges		
5 Cobras		6 Supermans		:30 Plank		
10 Jumping Jacks		10 Flutter Kicks		10 Toe Touches		
10 Toe Touches		4 Push-Ups		10 Marching Twists		
1:00 rest		1:00 rest		1:00 rest		
repeat		*repeat*		*repeat*		
20:00 evening walk		20:00 evening walk		20:00 evening walk		

Note: Warm up for 5 minutes prior to intervals or cross-training; stretch after each workout (cardio intervals, cross-training). See pages 135–39 for Warm-Ups & Stretches. Use exertion scale on page 76 for Easy, Moderate and Hard effort.

Prep Week 3 Running & Cross-Training

Mon	Tue	Wed	Thu	Fri	Sat	Sun
Morning: • 1:00 brisk walk • 1:00 normal walk *repeat 3x*	20:00 morning walk	Morning: • 1:00 brisk walk • 1:00 normal walk *repeat 3x*	30:00 morning walk	Morning: • 1:00 brisk walk • 1:00 normal walk *repeat 3x*	20:00 evening walk	Morning: • 10:00 normal walk • 10:00 brisk walk *repeat as many times as possible*
5:00 cool-down	6 Hip Raises	5:00 cool-down	6 Bird Dogs	5:00 cool-down		20:00 evening walk
20:00 evening walk	5 Squats	20:00 evening walk	4 Lunges	20:00 evening walk		
	6 Superman		:30 Plank			
	10 Flutter Kicks		4 Cobras			
	4 Push-Ups		10 Marching Twists			
	1:00 rest		1:00 rest			
	repeat		*repeat*			
	20:00 evening walk		20:00 evening walk			

Note: Warm up for 5 minutes prior to intervals or cross-training; stretch after each workout (cardio intervals, cross-training). See pages 135–39 for Warm-Ups & Stretches. Use exertion scale on page 76 for Easy, Moderate and Hard effort.

Prep Week 4 Running & Cross-Training

Mon	Tue	Wed	Thu	Fri	Sat	Sun
Morning: • 1:00 normal walk • 1:00 brisk walk • :30 jog *repeat 3x*	30:00 morning walk	Morning: • 1:00 normal walk • 1:00 brisk walk • :40 jog *repeat 3x*	30:00 morning walk	Morning: • 1:00 normal walk • 1:00 brisk walk • :50 jog *repeat 3x*	Morning: • 10:00 normal walk • 1:00 jog *repeat as many times as possible*	20:00 evening walk
5:00 cool-down	4 Hip Raises	5:00 cool-down	6 Mountain Climbers	5:00 cool-down	20:00 evening walk	
20:00 evening walk	4 Squats	20:00 evening walk	4 Lunges	20:00 evening walk		
	4 Supermans		:20 Plank			
	6 Flutter Kicks		8 Toe Touches			
	3 Push-Ups		8 Marching Twists			
	1:00 rest		1:00 rest			
	repeat sequence 2x		*repeat sequence 2x*			
	20:00 evening walk		20:00 evening walk			

Note: Warm up for 5 minutes prior to intervals or cross-training; stretch after each workout (cardio intervals, cross-training). See pages 135–39 for Warm-Ups & Stretches. Use exertion scale on page 76 for Easy, Moderate and Hard effort.

Prep Week 5 Running & Cross-Training

Mon	Tue	Wed	Thu	Fri	Sat	Sun
Morning: • 1:10 jog • :45 walk *repeat 3x*	Morning: • 10:00 normal walk • 10:00 brisk walk *repeat*	Morning: • 1:20 jog • :40 walk *repeat 3x*	Morning: • 10:00 normal walk • 10:00 brisk walk *repeat*	5:00 warm-up	20:00 evening walk	5:00 warm-up
5:00 cool-down	5 Hip Raises	5:00 cool-down	8 Mountain Climbers	Morning: • 1:30 jog • :30 walk *repeat 3x*		Morning: • 1:00 jog • :30 walk *repeat as many times as possible*
20:00 evening walk	5 Squats	20:00 evening walk	6 Lunges	5:00 cool-down		20:00 evening walk
	5 Cobras		4 Mason Twists	20:00 evening walk		
	4 In & Outs		6 Bird Dogs			
	4 Push-Ups		10 Marching Twists			
	1:00 rest		1:00 rest			
	repeat sequence 2x		*repeat sequence 2x*			
	20:00 evening walk		20:00 evening walk			

Note: Warm up for 5 minutes prior to intervals or cross-training; stretch after each workout (cardio intervals, cross-training). See pages 135–39 for Warm-Ups & Stretches. Use exertion scale on page 76 for Easy, Moderate and Hard effort.

Prep Week 6 Running & Cross-Training

Mon	Tue	Wed	Thu	Fri	Sat	Sun
1:40 jog	Morning: • 10:00 normal walk • 10:00 brisk walk *repeat*	Morning: • :30 jog • :20 walk *repeat 8x*	Morning: • 10:00 normal walk • 10:00 brisk walk *repeat*	Morning: • :40 jog • :20 walk *repeat 8x*	Morning: • 2:00 jog • 1:00 walk *repeat as many times as possible*	20:00 evening walk
:30 walk	6 Hip Raises	5:00 cool-down	8 Mountain Climbers	5:00 cool-down	5:00 cool-down	
repeat sequence 3x	5 Squats	20:00 evening walk	6 Lunges	20:00 evening walk	20:00 evening walk	
5:00 cool-down	4 In & Outs		4 Mason Twists			
20:00 evening walk	4 Push-Ups		10 Toe Touches			
	1:00 rest		10 Marching Twists			
	repeat sequence 2x		1:00 rest			
	20:00 evening walk		*repeat sequence 2x*			
			20:00 evening walk			

Note: Warm up for 5 minutes prior to intervals or cross-training; stretch after each workout (cardio intervals, cross-training). See pages 135–39 for Warm-Ups & Stretches. Use exertion scale on page 76 for Easy, Moderate and Hard effort.

Prep Week 7 Running & Cross-Training

Mon	Tue	Wed	Thu	Fri	Sat	Sun
Morning: • 2:10 jog • :40 walk *repeat 4x*	20:00 morning walk	Morning: • 2:20 jog • :40 walk *repeat 4x*	20:00 morning walk	Morning: • 2:20 jog • :30 walk *repeat 4x*	20:00 morning walk	Morning: • 2:30 jog • :30 walk *repeat as many times as possible*
5:00 cool-down	7 Hip Raises	5:00 cool-down	10 Mountain Climbers	5:00 cool-down	20:00 evening walk	5:00 cool-down
20:00 evening walk	6 Squats	20:00 evening walk	8 Lunges	20:00 evening walk		20:00 evening walk
	7 Cobras		6 Mason Twists			
	6 In & Outs		12 Toe Touches			
	5 Push-Ups		12 Marching Twists			
	1:00 rest		1:00 rest			
	repeat sequence 2x		*repeat sequence 2x*			
	20:00 evening walk		20:00 evening walk			

Prep to Level 1 Progression

Congratulations on completing the Prep Program! You've completed walk and jog intervals along with some serious cross-training to build your strength and running endurance. Take a moment to reflect on how far you've come in just seven weeks. You've run at least five minutes in a workout! With your daily walks, you have eclipsed over 100 miles of distance in less than two months!

Now, the work's not over yet. The goal to start the Level 1 Program is to be able to jog for at least 10 minutes at a time, and you may need to put in some time with the Prep Progression to get you there. We're going to drop the nightly walks in favor of starting off each day with slightly fresher legs to go longer. The cross-training workouts will also scale back to one session a week during this period, but don't worry, we'll hit it at full force again in the Level 1 Program. Repeat the Prep to Level 1 Progression as needed until you're able to hit 10:00 on the timer for your Sunday run. Don't worry if it takes you a few weeks even to complete the whole week. Take the progression as you need to in order to build up the strength and endurance you'll need to jump into the Level 1 Program.

Note: Warm up for 5 minutes prior to intervals or cross-training; stretch after each workout (cardio intervals, cross-training). See pages 135–39 for Warm-Ups & Stretches. Use exertion scale on page 76 for Easy, Moderate and Hard effort.

Prep Progression Running & Cross-Training

Mon	Tue	Wed	Thu	Fri	Sat	Sun
2:30 jog	rest	3:00 jog	10 Mountain Climbers	5:00 jog	rest	jog as long as possible
:10 walk		:10 walk	8 Lunges	:30 walk		5:00 cool-down
repeat sequence 3x		*repeat sequence 3x*	6 Mason Twists	*repeat sequence*		
5:00 cool-down		5:00 cool-down	8 Hip Raises	5:00 cool-down		
			10 Marching Twists			
			1:00 rest			
			repeat sequence 2x			

Level 1 Program

While it's called "Level 1," don't let the name fool you. This is an intense program designed to introduce and reinforce the core principles of building speed, strength and endurance. While the Prep Program is excellent for exposing new runners to building up their continuous running time as well as the many benefits of cross-training, the Level 1 Program will build on that foundation by adding jog/run intervals, tempo runs, pick-ups and hill repeats. The cross-training will get a little upgrade too, with two sessions a week composed of one full-body and one core-based routine to keep you limber while making you a stronger athlete that can withstand the rigors of high-intensity training. The stronger and more flexible you are, the more resistant to common injuries you'll be.

Who's the Level 1 Program good for?

- Experienced runners who are new to cross-training
- Runners who want to learn how to increase their distance
- Athletes looking to improve their speed
- Individuals who have a good level of fitness and are interested in bringing their performance and physique to the next level
- Runners of any distance looking for a new challenge

Level 1 Program requirements:

1. You need to be able to run for at least 10 minutes continuously, and should be right about at a mile in distance without stopping.

2. You should be familiar with bodyweight cross-training exercises like those in the Prep Program (page 88).

Want a good test? Follow the Prep to Level 1 Progression workout (page 100) for one week to assess your fitness level. If you get through all five workouts, you should be ready for the Level 1 Program, especially if you checked with your doctor first, right (see page 48)?

Since we're adding progressively longer runs throughout the program, it's important to note some key points:

- Every run is at your own pace, and initially that pace is just based upon your exertion scale and not a specific per-mile time. It's a relative pace and at your control; if you need to slow down or walk, that's totally up to you, bearing in mind that your goal is to complete the time or distance in the program.

- When the program calls for "easy," "moderate" or "hard" effort (see page 76 for descriptions), abide by it. There are specific intervals you'll reap benefits by running harder than others, but you'll get diminishing returns or risk overtraining injuries if you're constantly pushing the needle into the red. Follow the effort listed for each run.

- Back in "Interval Progression Training" on page 77, we covered the gamut of different types of running intervals we'll be performing in the Level 1 Program. In order to perform the workouts, you'll need to get familiar with these different drills or types of runs. Review the descriptions of jog/run intervals, tempo runs, pick-ups and hill repeats right now so you're ready to kick it into high gear in the following program. Performing these drills with the required set-up and intensity are critical to their effectiveness. Your knowledge of each and execution at the required intensity is what will set you apart from your fellow age groupers and make you fitter and faster than ever before.

Hill Repeats

You'll need a paved hill that's long enough for you to run up for at least 20 seconds, or up to 100 strides. A straight sidewalk, long driveway or safe side road will do. The hill doesn't need to be very steep (at least when you're just getting started) but should be enough of a bump to make a 20-second sprint up it a bit of a chore. Avoid grass, trails or stairs unless absolutely necessary as the focus of this drill is to build your running strength without worrying about footing, obstacles or tripping. Even if you're training for a trail race, this is a smooth-surface exercise; you can get your trail practice during your weekly mileage outside of these drills. Need to use a treadmill? See below.

The intervals are performed by running up the hill at the chosen level of exertion for the designed amount of time or number of strides. Once you hit that goal, slow, stop and turn around to descend the hill for the next repeat; walk or slow jog to return to the starting position. Don't dilly-dally, however; get back to the start for your next interval as quickly as you can while catching your breath. Hill repeats are quick, brutal and effective—the quicker you get them over with, the sooner you can rehydrate and move on with your workout.

Treadmill users: While you'll be missing out on the downhill walk or jog with each repetition, you can effectively use the treadmill to dial in a speed and incline that suits your ability and goals. Follow the appropriate warm-up of 5 minutes with the incline set at .5 or 1% and then carefully grab the handrails and step on the side rails while raising the incline to 5–10% based on your ability; change the speed so that you can safely maintain a moderate pace for the desired time. You'll need to adjust the incline and speed to hit your targets, so don't be afraid to carefully step off the belt if needed and make changes. When performing the intervals, run at the desired speed for the amount of time or strides in the program and then

carefully step off the belt onto the side rails to rest. Since you won't be walking or jogging downhill, take a 30-second to 1-minute break before your next interval, unless specifically instructed in the chart.

Pick-Ups

Understanding pick-up intervals is pretty easy; performing them is slightly more difficult. After warming up, you'll run for the specified distance or time at a designated pace or exertion level and then "pick up" your speed for an interval of time. Once your faster interval is over, return to the previous pace or exertion level and continue. If necessary, you may drop your intensity down to a walk for 30 seconds or so if you need to catch your breath, hydrate and recover.

Treadmill users should have no problem with this—just crank up the speed for the desired amount of time. The speed increase is relative to your ability and goals.

Tempo Runs

Tempo runs are defined as running for a prescribed period of time at a "hard" exertion level, or above 85% of your maximal effort or target heart rate (see "THR" on page 76). This pace is relative to your ability; as you progress it's a moving target. Keep that in mind when another runner shares their tempo pace or tries to tell you that it should be ANY exact minutes per mile. Your tempo is your tempo and will change from month to month based on your training. Got it?

Note: Warm up for 5 minutes prior to intervals or cross-training; stretch after each workout (cardio intervals, cross-training). See pages 135–39 for Warm-Ups & Stretches. Use exertion scale on page 76 for Easy, Moderate and Hard effort.

Level 1 Week 1 Running & Cross-Training

Mon	Tue	Wed	Thu	Fri	Sat	Sun
1-mi Easy Run	20 Jumping Jacks	1-mi Easy Run	8 Mason Twists	1-mi Easy Run	rest	25:00 jog (walk as needed)
1:00 walk/jog	12 Lunges	1:00 walk/jog	10 Hip Raises	1:00 walk/jog		5:00 cool-down
repeat	8 Push-Ups	*repeat*	8 Supermans	*repeat*		
5:00 cool-down	10 Mountain Climbers	5:00 cool-down	:40 Plank	5:00 cool-down		
	1:00 rest		1:00 rest			
	repeat sequence 2x		*repeat sequence 2x*			

Note: Warm up for 5 minutes prior to intervals or cross-training; stretch after each workout (cardio intervals, cross-training). See pages 135–39 for Warm-Ups & Stretches. Use exertion scale on page 76 for Easy, Moderate and Hard effort.

Level 1 Week 2 Running & Cross-Training

Mon	Tue	Wed	Thu	Fri	Sat	Sun
1.25-mi Easy Run	12 Marching Twists	1.25-mi Easy Run	:45 Side Plank (each side)	1.25-mi Easy Run	rest	25:00 jog (walk as needed)
1:00 walk/jog	6 Squats	1:00 walk/jog	10 Hip Raises	1:00 walk/jog		5:00 cool-down
repeat	8 Wood Chops	*repeat*	6 In & Outs	*repeat*		
5:00 cool-down	4 Inchworms	5:00 cool-down	12 Flutter Kicks	5:00 cool-down		
	1:00 rest		1:00 rest			
	repeat sequence 2x		*repeat sequence 2x*			

Note: Warm up for 5 minutes prior to intervals or cross-training; stretch after each workout (cardio intervals, cross-training). See pages 135–39 for Warm-Ups & Stretches. Use exertion scale on page 76 for Easy, Moderate and Hard effort.

Level 1 Week 3 Running & Cross-Training

Mon	Tue	Wed	Thu	Fri	Sat	Sun
1.25-mi Easy Run	20 Jumping Jacks	20/20 Drill (20 yd each): High Knees, Butt Kicks, Striders, Skips, Side Shuffle, Walking Lunges, Sprints, Backward Sprints	1:00 Plank	1.5-mi Easy Run	rest	35:00 jog (walk as needed)
1:00 walk/jog	12 Lunges	1:00 rest	10 Bicycle Crunches	1:00 walk/jog		5:00 cool-down
repeat	10 Push-Ups	*repeat*	10 Mason Twists	*repeat*		
5:00 cool-down	14 Mountain Climbers	5:00 cool-down	12 Superman	5:00 cool-down		
	1:00 rest		1:00 rest			
	repeat sequence 2x		*repeat sequence 2x*			

Note: Warm up for 5 minutes prior to intervals or cross-training; stretch after each workout (cardio intervals, cross-training). See pages 135–39 for Warm-Ups & Stretches. Use exertion scale on page 76 for Easy, Moderate and Hard effort.

Level 1 Week 4 Running & Cross-Training

Mon	Tue	Wed	Thu	Fri	Sat	Sun
1.5-mi Easy Run	6 Marching Twists	Hill Repeats • :20 Moderate intensity • :30 walk/jog *repeat 2x* • :20 Hard intensity • :30 walk *repeat 2x*	1:00 Plank	3-mi Easy Run	rest	45:00 jog (walk as needed)
:40 walk/jog	4 Squats	5:00 cool-down	8 Hip Raises	5:00 cool-down		5:00 cool-down
repeat	6 Wood Chops		8 In & Outs			
5:00 cool-down	3 Inchworms		8 Flutter Kicks			
	1:00 rest		1:30 rest			
	repeat sequence 3x		*repeat sequence 3x*			

Note: Warm up for 5 minutes prior to intervals or cross-training; stretch after each workout (cardio intervals, cross-training). See pages 135–39 for Warm-Ups & Stretches. Use exertion scale on page 76 for Easy, Moderate and Hard effort.

Level 1 Week 5 Running & Cross-Training

Mon	Tue	Wed	Thu	Fri	Sat	Sun
1.5-mi Easy Run	10 Box Jumps	Pick-Up Run: • 1-mi Easy • .5-mi Moderate • .25-mi Hard • 1:00 walk/jog *repeat*	8 Mason Twists	3-mi Moderate Run	rest	5-mi Easy Run
:30 walk/jog	8 Lunges		:30 Side Plank (each side)	5:00 cool-down		5:00 cool-down
repeat	5 Push-Ups		8 Supermans			
5:00 cool-down	14 Mountain Climbers		8 Bicycle Crunches			
	1:00 rest		1:00 rest			
	repeat sequence 3x		*repeat sequence 3x*			

Note: Warm up for 5 minutes prior to intervals or cross-training; stretch after each workout (cardio intervals, cross-training). See pages 135–39 for Warm-Ups & Stretches. Use exertion scale on page 76 for Easy, Moderate and Hard effort.

Level 1 Week 6 Running & Cross-Training

Mon	Tue	Wed	Thu	Fri	Sat	Sun
3-mi Easy Run	8 Marching Twists	2-mi Moderate/ Hard Tempo Run	1:00 Plank	3-mi Moderate Run	rest	6.2-mi Easy Run
5:00 cool-down	5 Squats	5:00 cool-down	8 Hip Raises	5:00 cool-down		5:00 cool-down
	8 Wood Chops	*repeat*	8 In & Outs			
	4 Inchworms		8 Flutter Kicks			
	1:00 rest		1:30 rest			
	repeat sequence 3x		*repeat sequence 3x*			

Note: Warm up for 5 minutes prior to intervals or cross-training; stretch after each workout (cardio intervals, cross-training). See pages 135–39 for Warm-Ups & Stretches. Use exertion scale on page 76 for Easy, Moderate and Hard effort.

Level 1 Week 7 Running & Cross-Training

Mon	Tue	Wed	Thu	Fri	Sat	Sun
3-mi Moderate Run	rest	3.5-mi Moderate/Hard Tempo Run	1:00 Plank	3.5-mi Moderate Run	rest	6.2-mi Easy Run
5:00 cool-down		5:00 cool-down	8 Hip Raises	5:00 cool-down		5:00 cool-down
		repeat	8 In & Outs			
			8 Flutter Kicks			
			1:30 rest			
			repeat sequence 3x			

After the Level 1 Program

Congratulations on completing the Level 1 Program. I sincerely hope you enjoyed it and are a faster, fitter runner! Are you ready for your first—or fastest—10K? If you haven't signed up already before starting the program, now's a great time to use your new level of training and fitness to totally stomp a new PR. Check out "Preparing for Your First Race" on page 140 to prepare you for the week leading up to and your first event.

If you're still in the quest for more fitness, strength and speed, then by all means step up to the challenge of the Level 2 Program. Bear in mind, the Level 1 Program may very well suit 80% of all runners looking to perform well in a 10K. The Level 2 Program is for extremely competitive athletes seeking to move up into the elite ranks and grab some age group or overall wins.

Level 2 Program

Congratulations on reaching the Level 2 Program! An overwhelming majority of athletes who pick up this book should start with the Prep and Level 1 Programs before jumping into this high-intensity seven-week workout routine. Building on the intervals and cross-training you learned in the earlier programs, this level is designed to push your limits of speed, strength and endurance. This program is intended to make the fit athlete even fitter, the fast runner even faster—it's not a beginner level in any way.

Remember back in "Before You Begin" on page 27 when I brought up how overtraining can absolutely sabotage your training with mental and physical fatigue? Well, if you're not an experienced runner who can complete at least 10 kilometers (6.2 miles) at a "hard" exertion level, this program is absolutely NOT designed for you to jump right into—at least not yet.

Assess your level: Complete the Level 1 Program first and after a week of taper, either race a 10K (optimal) or follow Week 6 of the Level 1 Program with all runs at moderate to hard intensity. If you're breezing through that workout, you're elite enough to step up to Level 2.

In addition to everything contained in the earlier programs, the Level 2 Program has cut the entire day of rest and replaced it with a full-body circuit and the 20/20 drill, and has also added a second "running session" drill as well. Just because you're working at a professional-athlete level doesn't mean that rest is less important— the exact opposite is true! In order to reap the benefits of this program, you need to get at least eight hours of solid, restful sleep a night and take it easy for the rest of the day before, between and after workouts (some days have two). Resist the temptation to add a 4000-yard swim session, play in a soccer league or race a Spartan Race, okay?

Who's the Level 2 Program good for?

- Extremely experienced runners looking to get fitter and faster in the least amount of time possible

- Professional and amateur athletes interested in developing extreme levels of conditioning in the off-season

Level 2 Program requirements:

1. You need to be able to run at medium to high intensity for at least 10 miles at a stretch without stopping.

2. You should be very familiar with bodyweight cross-training exercises like those found in the Level 1 Program, and be ready for 3–4 sessions a week on top of the required running regimen.

Back in "Interval Progression Training" on page 77, we covered the whole gamut of different types of running intervals we'll be performing in the Level 2 Program. You should've already learned how to perform jog/run intervals, tempo runs, pick-ups and hill repeats in the Level 1 Program, so you're ready to kick it into high gear in the following program. In the Level 2 Program we're going to add additional speed work to make you even faster. The cross-training routine also gets a jolt, moving to three days per week and incorporating some intensity in the form of supersets to continue to develop your strength and speed.

Speed Sessions

Short, intense runs above 90% of your maximal effort (THR) are what speed work is all about. An exertion level well into the "hard" range, speed work is designed for building your strength and speed (big surprise) through maintaining a pace for a brief interval just above lactate threshold (LT), or the point at which lactic acid begins to build up in your bloodstream. As you continue to perform speed work, your body will become more efficient at removing lactic acid from your bloodstream, thereby raising your LT.

Perform your speed work on a flat, paved surface or track to avoid any concerns about tripping over inconsistencies in the running surface or slipping on grass, dirt, etc. Run for the specified time or distance at the highest possible speed you can for each interval, slowing down to a stop or slow walk to rest in between sessions.

Treadmill users will find these similar to Hill Repeats, minus the incline change (stay at .5–1% incline) and for a longer period of time or distance. After your warm-up, crank the speed up to a pace that will push your heart rate to 90–95% of your maximum for the prescribed period of time. Carefully either lower the speed rapidly back down to a walking pace or grab on to the hand rails and step on the side rails during rest periods. Do I need to say "do this very carefully" again?

Note: Warm up for 5 minutes prior to intervals or cross-training; stretch after each workout (cardio intervals, cross-training). See pages 135–39 for Warm-Ups & Stretches. Use exertion scale on page 76 for Easy, Moderate and Hard effort.

Level 2 Week 1 Running & Cross-Training

Mon	Tue	Wed	Thu	Fri	Sat	Sun
2-mi Easy Run	20 Jumping Jacks	3-mi Hard Tempo Run	12 Marching Twists	3-mi Moderate Run	1:00 Plnk	6.2-mi Easy Run
2-mi Moderate Run	12 Lunges	5:00 cool-down	6 Squats	5:00 cool-down	10 Bicycle Crunches	5:00 cool-down
5:00 cool-down	8 Push-Ups		8 Wood Chops		10 Mason Twists	
	10 Mountain Climbers		4 Inchworms		12 Supermans	
	1:00 rest		1:00 rest		1:00 rest	
	repeat sequence 2x		*repeat sequence 2x*		:45 Side Plank (each side)	
	:45 Side Plank (each side)		1:00 Plank		10 Hip Raises	
	10 Hip Raises		10 Bicycle Crunches		6 In & Outs	
	4 In & Outs		10 Mason Twists		12 Flutter Kicks	
	12 Flutter Kicks		12 Supermans		1:00 rest	
	1:00 rest		1:00 rest		8 Bird Dogs	
	repeat sequence 2x		*repeat sequence 2x*		10 Mountain Climbers	
					6 Cobras	
					6 Child's Poses	
					1:00 rest	
					repeat sequence	

Note: Warm up for 5 minutes prior to intervals or cross-training; stretch after each workout (cardio intervals, cross-training). See pages 135–39 for Warm-Ups & Stretches. Use exertion scale on page 76 for Easy, Moderate and Hard effort.

Level 2 Week 2 Running & Cross-Training

Mon	Tue	Wed	Thu	Fri	Sat	Sun
20/20 Drill (20 yd each): High Knees, Butt Kicks, Striders, Skips, Side Shuffle, Walking Lunges, Sprints, Backward Sprints	1-mi Moderate Run	3-mi Hard Tempo Run	20 Jumping Jacks	Pick-Up Run: • 2-mi Easy • 2-mi Moderate • 1-mi Hard • 1-mi Easy • 1-mi Moderate	1:00 Plank	7-mi Easy Run
2:00 rest	1:00 rest	5:00 cool-down	12 Hip Raises	5:00 cool-down	10 Bicycle Crunches	5:00 cool-down
repeat	12 Marching Twists		8 Push-Ups		10 Mason Twists	
	6 Squats		10 Mountain Climbers		12 Supermans	
	10 Linear Reactive Step-Ups		1:00 rest		1:00 rest	
	10 Box Jumps		*repeat sequence 2x*		:45 Side Plank (each side)	
	1:00 rest		1:00 Plank		10 Hip Raises	
	repeat sequence		10 Bicycle Crunches		6 In & Outs	
			10 Mason Twists		12 Flutter Kicks	
			12 Supermans		1:00 rest	
			1:00 rest		8 Bird Dogs	
			repeat sequence 2x		10 Mountain Climbers	
					6 Cobras	
					6 Child's Poses	
					1:00 rest	
					repeat	

Note: Warm up for 5 minutes prior to intervals or cross-training; stretch after each workout (cardio intervals, cross-training). See pages 135–39 for Warm-Ups & Stretches. Use exertion scale on page 76 for Easy, Moderate and Hard effort.

Level 2 Week 3 Running & Cross-Training

Mon	Tue	Wed	Thu	Fri	Sat	Sun
20/20 Drill (20 yd each): High Knees, Butt Kicks, Striders, Skips, Side Shuffle, Walking Lunges, Sprints, Backward Sprints	1.5-mile Moderate Run	3.5-mile Hard Tempo Run	12 Marching Twists	Pick-Up Run: • 2-mi Easy • 2-mi Moderate • 1-mi Hard • 2-mi Easy • 1-mi Moderate	1:00 Plank	5-mi Moderate Run
2:00 rest	1:00 rest	5:00 cool-down	6 Squats	5:00 cool-down	10 Bicycle Crunches	5:00 cool-down
repeat sequence	20 Jumping Jacks		8 Wood Chops		10 Mason Twists	
	20 Hip Raises		4 Inchworms		12 Supermans	
	8 Push-Ups		1:00 rest		1:00 rest	
	10 Mountain Climbers		repeat sequence 2x		8 Bird Dogs	
	1:00 rest		10 Bicycle Crunches		10 Mountain Climbers	
	repeat sequence		10 Hip Raises		8 Cobras	
			10 Mason Twists		8 Child's Poses	
			12 Supermans		1:00 rest	
			1:00 rest		repeat sequence	
			repeat sequence 2x			

Note: Warm up for 5 minutes prior to intervals or cross-training; stretch after each workout (cardio intervals, cross-training). See pages 135–39 for Warm-Ups & Stretches. Use exertion scale on page 76 for Easy, Moderate and Hard effort.

Level 2 Week 4 Running & Cross-Training

Mon	Tue	Wed	Thu	Fri	Sat	Sun
20/20 Drill (20 yd each): High Knees, Butt Kicks, Striders, Skips, Side Shuffle, Walking Lunges, Sprints, Backward Sprints	1.5-mile Moderate Run	4-mile Hard Tempo Run	20 Jumping Jacks	Pick-Up Run: • 1-mi Easy • 2-mi Moderate • 1-mi Hard • 1-mi Easy • 1-mi Moderate	1:00 Plank	7-mi Moderate Run
2:00 rest	1:00 rest	5:00 cool-down	12 Hip Raises	5:00 cool-down	10 Bicycle Crunches	5:00 cool-down
12 Linear Reactive Step-Ups	12 Marching Twists		8 Push-Ups		10 Mason Twists	
14 Box Jumps	6 Squats		10 Mountain Climbers		12 Supermans	
1-mi Easy Run	10 Linear Reactive Step-Ups		1:00 rest		1:00 rest	
	10 Box Jumps		*repeat sequence 2x*		8 Bird Dogs	
	1:00 rest		1:00 Plank		10 Mountain Climbers	
	repeat sequence		10 Bicycle Crunches		6 Cobras	
			10 Mason Twists		6 Child's Poses	
			12 Supermans		1:00 rest	
			1:00 rest		*repeat sequence*	
			repeat sequence 2x			

Note: Warm up for 5 minutes prior to intervals or cross-training; stretch after each workout (cardio intervals, cross-training). See pages 135–39 for Warm-Ups & Stretches. Use exertion scale on page 76 for Easy, Moderate and Hard effort.

Level 2 Week 5 Running & Cross-Training

Mon	Tue	Wed	Thu	Fri	Sat	Sun
1-mile Moderate Run	Hill Repeats • :20 Moderate intensity • :30 Walk/Rest *repeat*	4-mi Hard Run	12 Marching Twists	Pick-Up Run: • 1-mi Easy • 2-mi Moderate • 1-mi Hard • 1-mi Easy • 1-mi Moderate	1:00 Plank	8-mi Moderate Run
1-mi Hard Run	Hill Repeats • :20 Hard intensity • :30 Walk/Rest *repeat 3x*	5:00 cool-down	6 Squats	5:00 cool-down	10 Bicycle Crunches	5:00 cool-down
1:00 rest	Hill Repeats • :20 Moderate intensity • :30 Walk/Rest *repeat 2x*	8 Bird Dogs	8 Wood Chops		10 Mason Twists	
20 Jumping Jacks	5:00 cool-down	10 Mountain Climbers	4 Inchworms		12 Supermans	
12 Hip Raises		6 Cobras	1:00 rest		1:00 Rest	
8 Push-Ups		6 Child's Poses	*repeat sequence 2x*		:45 Side Plank (each side)	
10 Mountain Climbers		1:00 rest	1:00 Plank		10 Hip Raises	
1:00 rest		*repeat sequence*	10 Bicycle Crunches		6 In & Outs	
repeat sequence			10 Mason Twists		12 Flutter Kicks	
			12 Supermans		1:00 rest	
			1:00 rest		8 Bird Dogs	
			repeat sequence 2x		10 Mountain Climbers	
					6 Cobras	
					6 Child's Poses	
					1:00 rest	
					repeat sequence	

Note: Warm up for 5 minutes prior to intervals or cross-training; stretch after each workout (cardio intervals, cross-training). See pages 135–39 for Warm-Ups & Stretches. Use exertion scale on page 76 for Easy, Moderate and Hard effort.

Level 2 Week 6 Running & Cross-Training

Mon	Tue	Wed	Thu	Fri	Sat	Sun
20-yd High Knees	1.5-mi Moderate Run	4-mi Hard Tempo Run	20 Jumping Jacks	Pick-Up Run: • 1-mi Easy • 1-mi Moderate • 1-mi Hard • 1-mi Easy • 1-mi Moderate • 1-mi Hard	1:00 Plank	5-mi Moderate/ Hard Run
20-yd Butt Kicks	1:00 rest	5:00 cool-down	12 Hip Raises	5:00 cool-down	10 Bicycle Crunches	5:00 cool-down
12 Linear Reactive Step-Ups	12 Marching Twist	8 Bird Dogs	8 Push-Ups		10 Mason Twists	
20-yd Strider	6 Squats	10 Mountain Climbers	10 Mountain Climbers		12 Supermans	
20-yd Skip	10 Linear Reactive Step-Ups	6 Cobras	1:00 rest		1:00 rest	
14 Box Jumps	10 Box Jumps	6 Child's Poses	*repeat sequence 2x*		:45 Side Plank (each side)	
20-yd Side Shuffle	1:00 rest	1:00 rest	1:00 Plank		10 Hip Raises	
20-yd Walking Lunges	*repeat sequence*	*repeat sequence*	10 Bicycle Crunches		6 In & Outs	
15 Push-Ups			10 Mason Twists		12 Flutter Kicks	
20-yd Sprint			10 Supermans		1:00 rest	
20-yd Backward Sprint			1:00 rest		8 Bird Dogs	
10 Mountain Climbers			*repeat sequence 2x*		10 Mountain Climbers	
1-mi Easy Run					6 Cobras	
					6 Child's Poses	
					1:00 rest	
					repeat sequence	

Note: Warm up for 5 minutes prior to intervals or cross-training; stretch after each workout (cardio intervals, cross-training). See pages 135–39 for Warm-Ups & Stretches. Use exertion scale on page 76 for Easy, Moderate and Hard effort.

Level 2 Week 7 Running & Cross-Training

Mon	Tue	Wed	Thu	Fri	Sat	Sun
2-mi Easy Run	20 Jumping Jacks	2-mi Easy Run	12 Marching Twists	4-mi Moderate Run	rest	6.2-mi Hard Run
3-mi Moderate Run	12 Lunges	3-mi Moderate Run	6 Squats	5:00 cool-down		5:00 cool-down
5:00 cool-down	8 Push-Ups	5:00 cool-down	8 Wood Chops			
	10 Mountain Climbers		4 Inchworms			
	1:00 rest		1:00 rest			
	repeat sequence 2x		*repeat sequence 2x*			
	:45 Side Plank (each side)		1:00 Plank			
	10 Hip Raises		10 Bicycle Crunches			
	6 In & Outs		10 Mason Twists			
	12 Flutter Kicks		12 Supermans			
	1:00 rest		1:00 rest			
	repeat sequence 2x		*repeat sequence 2x*			

After the Programs

Congratulations on completing the programs! Whether you found your groove with the Prep Program, progressed to Level 1 or even were up to the challenge of Level 2, I'm sincerely thrilled at your level of commitment to, and investment in, one of the most important elements of your life—developing a healthy, fit and sustainable lifestyle. Now that you've stuck with it through at least one program, you've proven to yourself that you can accomplish anything!

You can revisit these programs at any time to prepare for your next race. Whether you're looking to go farther or faster, you can use these workouts to continually progress and become a stronger, fitter runner.

APPENDIX

Functional Cross-Training Exercises

Squat

Squat form is crucial to getting the most out of this extremely beneficial exercise. Check out your form by using a full-body mirror and standing perpendicular to it as you complete your reps.

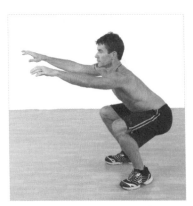

1 Stand tall with your feet shoulder-width apart and toes pointed slightly outward. Raise your arms until they're parallel to the floor.

2 Bend at the hips and knees and "sit back" as if you were about to sit down into a chair. Keep your head up, eyes forward and arms out in front of you for balance. As you descend, contract your glutes while your body leans forward slightly so that your shoulders are almost in line with your knees. Your knees should not extend past your toes; do not roll up on the balls of your feet. Stop when your thighs are parallel to the floor.

Push straight up from your heels to stand. Don't lock your knees at the top of the exercise.

Lunge with Twist

This movement is exactly like a forward or reverse lunge, but your hands and core can get in on the fun.

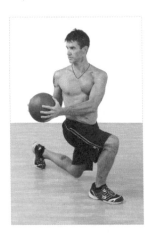

1 Stand tall with your feet shoulder-width apart and both hands on opposite sides of a medicine ball, elbows slightly bent.

2 Keeping the ball in front of you, step forward (or backward) with your right foot to start the lunge. As you lower your hips, twist your core and swing the ball laterally to your right until both knees are bent 90° and your arms are extended and holding the medicine ball to the right, 90° from where you started.

Return to the start. Repeat to the other side.

Marching Twist

Start slowly and work up the intensity.

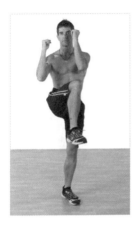

1 Stand tall with your feet shoulder-width apart. Bring your arms in front of you and bend your elbows 90°.

2 Twist your torso to the right and raise your right knee to your left elbow.

3 Repeat with your left knee and right elbow. A little hop with the bottom foot helps you keep your momentum going from leg to leg.

Jumping Jacks

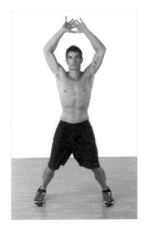

1 Stand tall with your feet together and arms extended along your sides, palms facing forward.

2 Jump 6–12 inches off the ground and simultaneously spread your feet apart an additional 20–30 inches while extending your hands directly overhead.

Jump 6–12 inches off the ground and return your hands and feet to start position.

Wood Chop

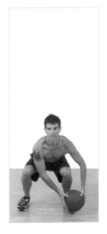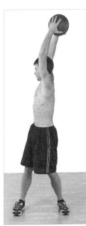

1 Stand tall with your feet shoulder-width apart, holding a medicine ball in front of you.

2 Lower your body into a squat until your knees are bent 90°, and bring the ball down to touch your left foot.

3 Stand tall, twisting your torso to the right and lifting your arms straight up over your head. Your left shoulder should be in front and you should be looking to the right.

Repeat to the other side.

MODIFICATION: This can also be done without a medicine ball.

Linear Reactive Step-Up

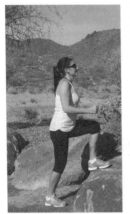
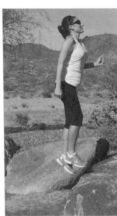

1 Stand 12–18 inches in front of a bench or object 18–24 inches tall that can hold your weight; have your hands at your sides and feet shoulder-width apart.

2 Step up with your left foot and place it flat on top of the bench, leaving your right foot on the ground.

3 Push down with your left foot and jump up as high as you can using only the strength of your left leg. Your right leg should not be pushing off at all. Let your arms swing naturally at your sides as you jump.

4 Switch legs in mid-air by bringing your left foot backward and right foot forward at the apex of your jump. Your right foot will land on top of the bench and your left foot on the ground.

As soon as your right foot lands on the bench, immediately jump again using only the strength of your right leg. That's 2 reps.

Box Jump

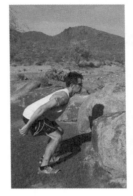
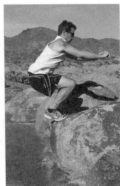

1 Stand 12–18 inches in front of a box or bench that's 24–36 inches tall and can hold your weight. Keep your hands at your sides and feet shoulder-width apart.

2 Initiate the jump by dropping your hips and bending at the waist in a squat movement, but only about half as deep. Swing your arms back and shift your weight toward the front of your feet.

Inchworm

In this motion-based exercise, you'll advance forward approximately 4 feet per repetition, so plan your exercise positioning accordingly.

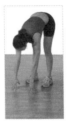
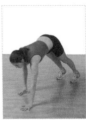
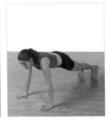

1 Stand with your feet about hip-width apart and fold over so that your hands touch the floor.

2 Keeping your hands firmly on the floor to balance your weight, walk your hands out in front of you one at a time until you're at the top of a push-up. Hold for 3 seconds.

3 Keeping your hands firmly on the floor to balance your weight, "walk" your feet toward your head by taking very small steps on your toes (imagine that your lower legs are bound together and you can only bend your feet at each ankle). Your butt will rise and your body will form an inverse "V." When you've stretched your hamstrings, glutes and calves as far as you can, hold that position for 3 seconds.

Mountain Climbers

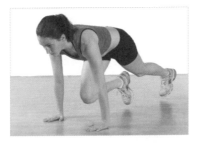

1 Assume the top position of a push-up with your hands directly under your shoulders and toes on the ground. Keep your core engaged and your body in a straight line from head to toe.

2 Lift your right toe slightly off the ground, bring your right knee to your chest and place your right foot on the ground under your body.

3 With a very small hop from both toes, extend your right foot back to starting position and at the same time bring your left knee to your chest and place your left foot on the ground under your body.

Continue switching, making sure to keep your hips low.

Push-Up

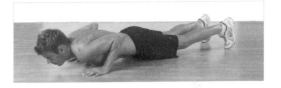

1 Place your hands on the ground approximately shoulder-width apart, making sure your fingers point straight ahead and your arms are straight but your elbows not locked. Step your feet back until your body forms a straight line from head to feet. Your feet should be about 6 inches apart. Engage your core to keep your spine from sagging; don't sink into your shoulders.

2 Inhale as you lower your torso to the ground and focus on keeping your elbows as close to your sides as possible, stopping when your elbows are at 90° or your chest is 1–2 inches from the floor.

Push your torso back up to starting position.

Plank

The plank is exactly like the top portion of a push-up.

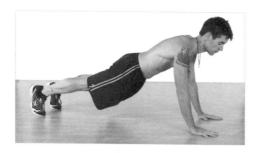

Place your hands on the ground approximately shoulder-width apart, making sure your fingers point straight ahead and your arms are straight but your elbows not locked. Step your feet back until your body forms a straight line from head to feet. Your feet should be about 6 inches apart. Engage your core to keep your spine from sagging; don't sink into your shoulders and don't let your butt sag. Once you can no longer keep your back flat, lower yourself to the floor.

Side Plank

The side plank is a great isolation exercise for tightening your internal and external abdominal obliques (aka your love handles) as well as the transverse abdominis.

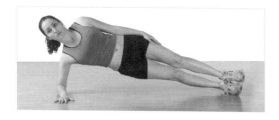

1 Lie on your side and stack your feet, hips and shoulders atop each other. Prop yourself up on your elbow, keeping it directly under your shoulder; your forearm should be completely on the ground, perpendicular to your body.

2 Engaging your core to keep your spine erect, lift your hips off the floor until you form a nice line from head to feet. Let your top arm rest along your side. Hold the position for a predetermined amount of time or for as long as possible.

Slowly lower your hips to the floor. Repeat on the opposite side.

MODIFICATION: If you have weak knees, you can use a foam roller, medicine ball or similar to provide some knee joint stability. Place the object on the outside of the thigh that is closest to the ground and keep your legs straight. You may need to experiment with the positioning to get comfortable.

Hip Raise

This exercise is a slow and controlled motion that works the entire core—back, hips and abs—and provides a great way to work those muscles without any impact.

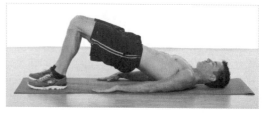

1 Lie on your back with your knees bent and feet flat on the floor, as close to your butt as possible. Place your arms and palms flat on the floor at your sides.

2 Engage your abdominal muscles and exhale while you press your feet into the floor and raise your hips and lower back up, forming a straight line from your sternum to your knees. Do not push your hips too high or arch your back. Hold for 3–5 seconds, and then inhale and slowly return to start.

Superman

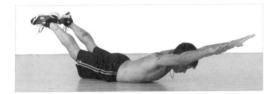

1 Lying face down on your stomach, extend your arms directly out in front of you and your legs behind you. Keep your knees straight as if you were flying.

2 In a slow and controlled manner, contract your erector spinae and raise your arms and legs about 6–8 inches off the floor. Hold for 5 seconds.

Lower yourself slowly.

Flutter Kick

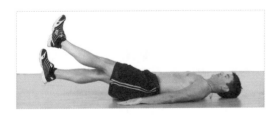

1 Lie flat on your back with your legs extended along the floor and your arms along your sides, palms down.

2 Contract your lower abdominal muscles and lift your feet 6 inches off the floor. Hold for 5 seconds.

3 While keeping your left foot in place, lift your right foot 6 inches higher (it should now be 12 inches off the floor). Hold for 5 seconds.

4 Simultaneously lower your right leg back to 6 inches off the floor while raising your left foot 6 inches higher. Hold for 5 seconds.

This counts as 2 reps.

Bicycle Crunch

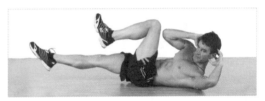

1 Lie flat on your back with your legs extended straight along the floor and your hands at both sides of your head, fingers touching your temples. Raise your feet 6 inches off the floor while simultaneously contracting your abs and lifting your upper back and shoulders off the floor.

2 In one movement, bend your left knee and raise your left leg so that the thigh and shin are 90°; rotate your torso using your oblique muscles so that your right elbow touches the inside of your left knee.

3 Rotate your torso back to center and lower your upper body toward the floor, stopping before your shoulders touch.

4 Extend your left knee and return your foot to 6 inches off the floor and bend your right leg 90°. Contract your abs, rotate, and touch your left elbow to the inside of your right knee.

That's 2 reps.

Mason Twist

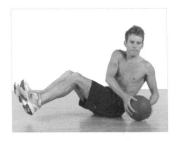

1 Sit on the floor with your knees comfortably bent, feet on the floor, arms bent 90° and hands holding a medicine ball or weight in front of your chest.

2 Lift your feet about 4–6 inches off the floor and balance your body weight on your posterior. Keep your core tight to protect your back. While maintaining the same hip position, twist your entire torso at the waist and touch the ball to the floor on the left side of your body.

3 Keeping your feet off the floor and maintaining your balance, rotate back to center and then to your right to touch the ball to the floor.

Return to center. This is 1 rep.

In & Out

Aside from planks, this is my favorite core move due to its full range of motion and how well it works the entire rectus abdominis and erector spinae without putting excessive force on your upper spine and neck. This is a very slow and controlled motion and is performed best at a cadence of 3 seconds in, 3 seconds hold and 3 seconds out.

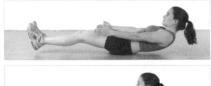

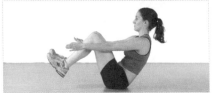

1 Lie flat on your back with your legs extended straight along the floor and your arms along your sides, palms down.

2 Lift your feet about 3 inches off the floor, bend your knees and bring your feet toward your butt while simultaneously lifting your arms off the floor and activating your abs to roll your upper body upward.

3 Continue raising your head and shoulders off the floor and bringing your hands past the outside of your knees while bringing your knees and chest together. At the top of the move, pause for 1–3 seconds.

Slowly return to starting position. Be careful to "roll" your spine in a natural movement and let your shoulders and head lightly touch the floor.

Cobra

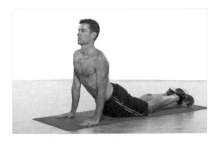

Lying on your stomach, place your hands directly under your shoulders with your fingers forward; straighten your legs and point your toes. Exhale while lifting your chest off the floor and pushing your hips gently into the floor. Your arms help guide you through the movement; your elbows should remain slightly bent at the top of the extension and your hips should remain in contact with the floor. Hold for 15–30 seconds and then gently roll your upper body back to the floor.

Bird Dog

The bird dog is an excellent exercise for developing abdominal and hip strength and flexibility, and also for working your lower back.

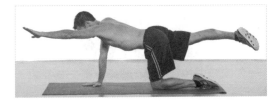

1 Get on your hands and knees with your knees bent 90° and under your hips, toes on the floor and your hands on the floor directly below your shoulders. Keep your head and spine neutral; do not let your head lift or sag. Contract your abs to prevent your back from sagging; keep your back flat for the entire exercise.

2 In one slow and controlled motion, simultaneously raise your right leg and left arm until they're on the same flat plane as your back. Your leg should be parallel to the ground, not raised above your hip; your arm should extend directly out from your shoulder and your biceps should be level with your ear. Hold this position for 3–5 seconds and then slowly lower your arm and leg back to starting position.

Toe Touch

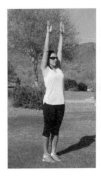 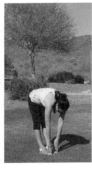

1 Stand with your feet approximately shoulder-width apart and back straight. Lift your arms directly above your head with your palms facing forward. Reach up as high as you can.

2 Hinge at your waist and, keeping your arms overhead and back as straight as possible, lower your upper torso as one unit to bring your head toward your knees. Try to touch your toes with your fingertips. Do not bounce or grab your ankles in an attempt to pull your upper body farther down. Hold in the down position for 5 seconds.

Slowly return to starting position with your arms extended over your head.

Repeat, each subsequent time trying to stretch a little farther than the previous repetition.

20/20 Series

The 20/20 Drill combines eight moves at high intensity to develop your speed, strength, agility, endurance and all-around athletic ability. This drill is short and intense as a workout, and also provides a great warm-up and cool-down when performed at a more-relaxed pace.

Find a flat area at least 20 yards long and place some cones or markers at each end; pavement or grass is fine, a sports field is optimal. Perform each of the following movements back to back with little or no rest in between. Perform the first exercise/movement for 20 yards until you reach your marker, turn around and perform the next exercise/movement 20 yards back to the starting point, continually progressing through all eight moves at a high intensity, with good form and little to no rest in between.

High Knees

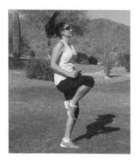

Run forward using a normal-length stride. Bend the knee of your elevated leg 90° and raise it

until it's level with your waist. Push forward from the ball of your grounded foot, switch legs, and repeat. Pump your arms to generate leg drive and speed.

Butt Kicks

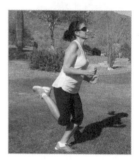

Run forward by taking very small steps and raising the heel of your back leg up toward your buttocks. Push forward from the ball of your grounded foot, progressing 12–18 inches per stride.

Striders

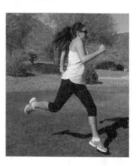

Bound forward by pushing off hard from the ball of your grounded foot, pumping your arms to generate leg drive and speed. Take huge leaps forward, trying to cover as much ground as possible with each stride.

Skip

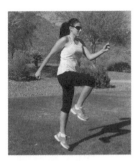

Bound forward by pushing off hard from the ball of your grounded foot, landing again on that same foot and pushing off once more before landing on the opposite foot. Pump your arms to generate leg drive and speed. Take smaller leaps forward than when performing Striders, covering slightly less ground per stride.

Side Shuffle

Turn sideways with your left hip pointing toward the direction you'll be traveling, feet slightly wider than your shoulders and hands at your sides. Push off with your right foot in the direction you'll be traveling while lifting your left foot and swinging your right foot toward the center of your body. Touch both feet together lightly before landing on your right foot, extending your left foot out to the side in the direction you're traveling and repeating the process. *When you reach the 10-yard mark, turn 180 degrees so that your right hip is pointing in the direction that you're traveling and continue side shuffling an additional 10 yards.*

Walking Lunge

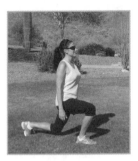

Stand tall, facing the direction you'll be traveling, with your feet shoulder-width apart and your arms hanging at your sides. Take a large step forward with your right foot, bend both knees and drop your hips straight down until both knees are bent 90°. Your left knee should almost be touching the ground and your left toes are on the ground behind you. Keep your core engaged and your back, neck and hips straight at all times during this movement. Keeping your right foot in place on the ground, push up with your right leg, straighten both knees, bring your left leg parallel with your right, and place your left foot next to your right. Continue moving forward by repeating the above process with your left foot.

Backward Sprint

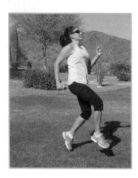

Facing away from the direction you'll be traveling, run by pushing off alternating forefeet and raising your knees as high as possible. Pump your arms as needed to generate leg drive and speed. This takes a little getting used to but it's a great way to strengthen your running muscles by working them in an opposite plane of motion. It also helps to develop balance and agility.

Sprint

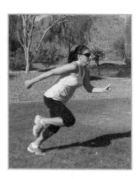

The sprint is saved for last so you're working extremely hard to generate speed after your legs and lungs are already fatigued. Run forward at top speed by leaning forward with your upper body to as much as a 45° angle and driving off the balls of your feet as hard and as rapidly as you can. Pump your arms to increase leg drive and speed.

Warming Up

Properly warming up the body prior to any activity is very important, as is stretching post-workout to kick-start recovery by loosening up the muscles to allow optimal blood flow. Please note that warming up and stretching are two completely different things: A warm-up routine should be done before stretching so that your muscles are more pliable and able to be stretched efficiently. You should not "warm up" by stretching; you simply don't want to push, pull or stretch cold muscles.

It's crucial to raise your body temperature prior to beginning a workout. In order to prevent injury, such as a muscle strain, you want to loosen up your muscles and joints before you begin any rapid movements. A good warm-up before your workout should slowly raise your core body temperature, heart rate and breathing.

Before jumping into the workout, you must increase blood flow to all working areas of the body. This augmented blood flow will transport more oxygen and nutrients to the muscles being worked. The warm-up will also increase the range of motion of your joints.

Luckily for you, walking and jogging are excellent ways to warm up prior to a running or cross-training workout. A 5- to 10-minute progression from a casual walk to a brisk walk followed by a slow, easy jog will do the trick. Once you're warm and at a safe place to perform some dynamic stretches, follow the 5-minute program below to prepare you for a great workout or race.

"Poor Man's Yoga" Dynamic Warm-Up

Be sure to perform each movement carefully and correctly to maximize the benefits. Never bounce or yank with your arms to pull yourself into the head-to-knees position. As you repeat, each subsequent movement should provide a little deeper range of motion.

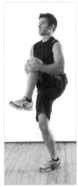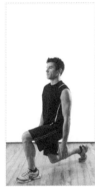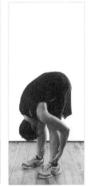

1 In one controlled, sequential movement, stand up straight, bring one knee to your chest.

2 Release and step into a forward lunge.

3 Then step forward with your opposite foot and stand straight up, bend at the waist and lower your head to your knees while keeping your knees straight. Place your hands on the backs of your lower calves and pull slightly to assist in getting your noggin closer to your knees.

4 Release your hands, slowly return to standing and then carefully roll your weight up to the balls of both feet. Keeping your body in an athletic position, extend your feet using your calves to slowly raise your bodyweight straight up. Keep your balance and hold the extended position for 3 seconds, then slowly lower your heels to the floor.

That's 1 rep; repeat with your right leg. Perform 5 reps on each side.

Side-to-Side Leg Swing

1 Stand facing a wall about 2 feet away.

2 Lean forward slightly, extend your arms forward and place your hands against the wall to support your weight.

3 Lift your right foot off the ground and maintain your balance while lifting up on the toes of your left foot. Swing your right leg in front of your left and then out to the right in a pendulum motion while keeping your knee straight. Continue swinging your leg for 10–15 seconds to loosen your right hip and glutes, gradually making an increasingly larger arc with your leg. Switch legs and repeat.

Front-to-Back Leg Swing

1 Stand facing a wall about two feet away. Turn 90° so that the wall is to your right and place your right hand on the wall.

2 Lift your right foot off the ground. Maintain your balance while lifting up on the toes of your left foot and swing your right leg in an arc in front of you with your knee straight and then swing it back behind you, bending your knee to bring your heel close to your buttocks. Continue swinging your leg for 10–15 seconds, gradually increasing the size of your arc.

Turn to your left side, place your left hand on the wall and repeat with your left leg.

20/20 Warm-Up Drill

In the Level 1 and Level 2 Programs, we covered variations of the 20/20 Drill to build strength, speed, flexibility and stamina. A few of them are a fantastic way to warm your legs, hips and glutes up before a run. Since they're a warm-up, not a workout, keep the intensity low and progress through each of the following moves.

:15–:30 Butt Kicks (page 132)

:15–:30 Striders (page 132)

:15–:30 High Knees (page 132)

:15–:30 Skip (page 133)

Jog for 2 minutes to keep warm and loosen up any tight muscles you may have.

Arm Circle

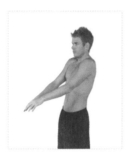

1 Stand with your feet shoulder-width apart.

2 Move both arms in a complete circle forward 5 times and then backward 5 times.

Side Bend

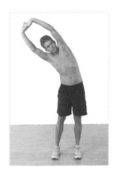

Stand with your feet shoulder-width apart and extend your hands overhead with elbows locked, fingers interlocked and palms up. Bend side to side.

Lumber Jack

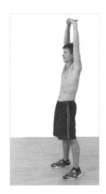 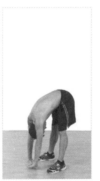

1 Stand with your feet shoulder-width apart and extend your hands overhead with elbows locked, fingers interlocked and palms up.

2 Bend forward at the waist and try to put your hands on the ground (like you're chopping wood). Raise up and repeat.

Around the World

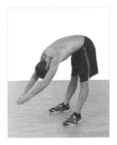

1 Stand with your feet shoulder-width apart and extend your hands overhead with elbows locked, fingers interlocked and palms up. Keep your arms straight the entire time.

2 Bending at the hips, bring your hands down toward your right leg and in a continuous circular motion bring your hands toward your toes, then toward your left leg, and then return your hands overhead and bend backward. Repeat 3 times, then change directions.

Stretches

After your workout, stretching will help you reduce soreness from the workout, increase range of motion and flexibility within a joint or muscle, and prepare your body for any future workouts. Stretching immediately post-exercise while your muscles are still warm allows your muscles to return to their full range of motion (which gives you more flexibility gains) and reduces the chance of injury or fatigue in the hours or days after an intense workout.

Remember: Even when you're warm and loose, never "bounce" during stretching. Keep your movements slow and controlled. The stretches in this section should be performed in order to optimize your recovery. Remember to exhale as you perform every deep stretch and rest 30 seconds in between each stretch.

Forearm & Wrist

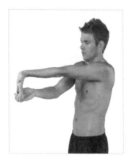

Stand with your feet shoulder-width apart and extend both arms straight out in front of you. Keep your back straight. Turn your right wrist to the sky and grasp your right fingers from below with your left hand. Slowly pull your fingers back toward your torso with your left hand; hold for 10 seconds.

Swap arms and repeat.

Shoulders

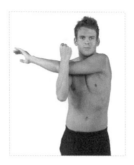

Stand with your feet shoulder-width apart and bring your left arm across your chest. Support your left elbow with the crook of your right arm by raising your right arm to 90°. Gently pull your left arm to your chest while maintaining a straight back and wide shoulders. Don't round or hunch your shoulders. Hold for 10 seconds. Release and switch arms. After you've done both sides, shake your hands out for 5 to 10 seconds.

Shoulders & Upper Back

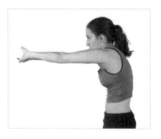

1 Stand with your feet shoulder-width apart and extend both arms straight out in front of you. Interlace your fingers and turn your palms to face away from your body. Keep your back straight.

2 Exhale and push your palms straight out from your body by pushing through your shoulders and upper back. Allow your neck to bend naturally as you round your upper back. Continue to reach your hands and stretch for 10 seconds.

Rest for 30 seconds then repeat. After you've done the second set, shake your arms out for 10 seconds to your sides to return blood to the fingers and forearm muscles.

Chest & Arms

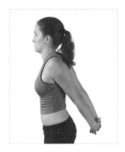

Clasp your hands together behind your lower back with palms facing each other. Keeping an erect posture and your arms as straight as possible, gently pull your arms away from your back, straight out behind you. Keep your shoulders down. Hold for 10 seconds.

Rest for 30 seconds and repeat.

Child's Pose

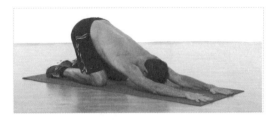

From a kneeling position, sit your buttocks back on your calves then lean forward and place your lower torso on your thighs. Extend your arms directly out in front of you, parallel to each other, and lower your chest toward the floor. Reach your arms as far forward as you can and rest your forearms and hands flat on the floor. Hold for 30 seconds.

FOAM ROLLER RELEASE

Entire books have been written about using a foam roller to reduce muscle soreness, return blood flow, loosen fascia and massage deep-tissue; there's no way to cover them all in this book. What I do recommend is following some of the simple instructions that can be found with most any foam roller that you purchase from a local sport's store or online—make sure whichever one you purchase comes with some example stretches and recovery techniques to get you started. Most commonly, you'll support your bodyweight on top of the roller with it under your glutes, hamstrings, quads, IT band, hips and back in order to give your muscles a deep massage. If you need some tips on models I recommend, check out my "Gear" section on www.7weekstofitness.com.

Preparing for Your First Race

I was once told this little nugget of wisdom from an experienced runner: "You're not going to get any faster the week before a race—you can only end up hurting yourself." This is the reason that runners need to limit their running distance and intensity for 7–10 days leading up to a race. In order to run your best, you'll need to be rested and ready, not tired and sore. If you're following the Level 1 or Level 2 programs, make sure you have at least a week between the last workout and your event. During that week, you still need to run a bit in order to stay loose, so cut your training down to 50% intensity at 50% of the distance. For example, the final week of the Level 1 Program is six days of training, logging approximately 25 miles of running at varying intensity. Your taper week will consist of 3 runs of 4 miles at 50% intensity. Cool?

Race Day

Remember your goals, how far you've come and relax. Enjoy the moment, soak in your first race and learn from the experience. Really, it's that simple. You're guaranteed a PR—it's your first race! Setting any type of time goal for your first race can lead to disaster as you've never been here before. Take the race seriously, but make sure you have some fun and you may just be pleasantly surprised when you see your finish time.

Lay all your clothes and gear out the night before. If you've already attended the race expo then make sure you have your bib number and timing chip (if your event is using them). Set your alarm early for race day—you'll need time to wake up, grab a cup of coffee (if that's your thing), shower, hit the restroom as many times as you need and get to your event with plenty of time to spare. Parking can be a bit of a mess with street closures, so plan for taking an alternate route around the course. Most large events will provide a pretty comprehensive map of the start area showing where parking, port-o-potties and the start corrals are located. When driving, parking and walking to the start area, you can usually get by following other runners. The same holds true for the race—you probably won't be in first place (okay, you won't) so even on poorly marked courses, as long as you can keep other runners in sight, you're A-OK.

A little planning goes a long way, and it starts with researching the event online. Note the course, water stations and elevation change by reviewing the event's map, but also make sure you know where the port-o-potties, starter corrals, and bag drop (if the event has one) are before you show up on race day. It's your responsibility to know everything from the proper course to the rules; know the specifics and manage your day effectively.

Tip: Plan a spot to meet your running partners before the event and where to locate them as well as friends and family after the race. In the busy, loud and bustling area after the finish line, it can be nearly impossible to spot your crew. Add in a hefty dose of elation and fatigue and you can spend hours wandering around

RACE-DAY CHECKLIST

❏ Fresh socks, worn in but not threadbare

❏ Anti-chafe

❏ Sunglasses

❏ Broken-in (not broken-down) shoes

❏ Pre-race drink for hydration, energy and electrolytes (or water and electrolyte tablets)

❏ Snack or energy gel

❏ Warm/comfy pre- and post-race clothes, sandals, etc.

❏ Watch, heart rate monitor or other gizmos (leave the music behind, see page 35)

❏ Race belt or number bib and safety pins (see "Race Belt" below)

❏ Event's timing chip (if applicable)

❏ Sunscreen, visor

❏ Gear "drop" bag (if applicable)

❏ Weather-appropriate running clothes: gloves, hat, arm warmers, tights

❏ Post-race recovery food or drink

A printable version of this checklist is available on www.7weekstofitness.com.

searching the crowd. If you orchestrate your meet-up point well, your spectators can bring some adequate post-race nutrition and a change of clothes. The less you have to put into your bag drop, the better.

USING THE BAG DROP

Large, longer-distance events like a half or full marathon will usually have a bag drop, but a growing number of 5K and 10Ks are starting to as well. Racers can pick up a drop bag with their race packet (usually a race bib, timing chip, race-day info and some product samples or coupons from sponsors) and deposit it in a specified location before the start of the race. Useful for storing a post-race snack or depositing your pre-race warm clothes into before the race, these bags should never carry anything valuable, like a cell phone, jewelry or car keys. Bags commonly get crushed, lost or even wet if other racers put drinks in their bags, so remember that you've been warned.

In order to limit the stress on race day, here are some tips to keep in mind when using a gear check or drop bag:

- Don't put any valuables into a drop bag.
- Leave your cell phone in your car. Don't count on technology to find your friends

TIP: While most races will have bananas, bagels or sports drinks after the finish, it's usually up to you to bring a snack with adequate protein to kick-start your recovery. Put a sports bar in your drop bag and even ask your spectators to bring one along for you.

and family—pick a spot to meet up at in a specified time range.

- Do put a snack like a nutrition bar with carbs and protein to aid recovery.
- Do not put a drink in your drop bag unless you want it to leak all over your—and everyone else's—stuff.
- Don't leave your car keys in the drop bag. If it gets lost then you're really stuck. Take the door key or remote–not the whole key ring–along with you or hide it somewhere under your car.
- Tie a brightly colored ribbon on your bag. It will make it easier to spot in the pile and you can tell the volunteer, "It's the one with the Hello Kitty bow on it."

The Starting Line

Make sure you get to your designated starting corral in time for the gun. This comes from someone who has missed a few starts in his day while in the port-o-potty, getting stuck in traffic or standing with the wrong group of runners (I was with the 5K start, not the 10K group nearly two football fields away, and missed the start by over a minute!).

When the starter yells "GO!" make sure you keep your bubbling emotions in check; start out slow and find a comfortable pace. It may take you a while to find your rhythm—feel free to let anyone pass if they want to run faster. If you're in a race that doesn't have time-specific corrals, then position yourself near the back and concentrate on running your own race—don't worry about anyone else!

WHAT'S A RACE OR HYDRATION BELT?

One of the simplest and cheapest pieces of equipment for race day that can really make an impact is a race belt. An adjustable, stretchy band of material with a closure and some snaps to hold your number bib, a race belt provides a serviceable place for you to affix your number without having to pin it to your shirt or shorts. A race belt also allows you to change the positioning of your number as you run and even remove layers of clothing as temperatures and conditions change. Some race belts can feature small enclosures for a key, energy bar or gel, while larger ones, usually referred to as hydration belts, provide options to carry flasks along on your run.

A multibottle hydration belt is best suited for long training runs that are over an hour as the more liquid you carry, the heavier you'll be. As most races provide water or sports drink about every one to two miles on the course, filling up a multi-bottle hydration belt may make you feel a little bit like a pack mule, and surely not as fast and light as you'd want during a timed race! If you want to carry a drink, limit it to a single, small four- to six-ounce flask. A modular hydration belt will make this possible by sliding off the unneeded bottle holders.

Tip: While it's always smart to "be prepared," you don't necessarily need to carry an entire snack bar and load of gizmos around your waist during an event. There's no prize for the guy or gal running around with Batman's utility belt. Unless you have extreme energy requirements, three to four energy gels are more than enough for any marathon, as nearly all events will provide them at least a couple times on-course. One caveat: In a self-supported race, it's up to you to carry everything you may need, and there's no aid provided on-course. Consider a self-supported race like a training run of similar distance and bring along at least the minimum required hydration and nutrition you would use in training—and possibly a little more if you can carry it.

Race or hydration belts without pockets still make it possible to pin, tape or wrap an elastic to keep a gel or two in an accessible area on your waist. Just make sure the weight of any gels doesn't drag the belt down as you run!

Navigating the Water Stations

There's no denying that water stations can be utter chaos in bigger events, with folks diving in front of you, wet pavement and cups everywhere and even the occasional oblivious runner who stops dead right in front of people. Here's how to handle each aid station effectively:

Pick one of the last volunteers, shoot for one three-quarters from the end of the station so even if you miss their cup you can grab another. If you're planning to walk a little bit at each water station (a great plan for first-timers, by the way), make sure you're past the aid station and there are no runners directly behind you. Slow down gradually and pull over to the side of the road and walk briskly while you catch your breath and hydrate.

Even if you choose to keep running, it's important for you to learn how to drink out of a cup on the run, a skill that you most likely never practice in training with your nice little pop-top water bottle. When the volunteer holds out the water cup, reach out, make soft contact with the cup and then absorb some of the contact so you don't snatch the cup out of their hand, causing you both a little shower and wasting the water you're looking forward to drinking. Once you have the cup, pinch your index finger and thumb together from opposite sides of the cup near the top rim—this will form a little spout that will help you direct the water into your mouth a little more easily.

Take small sips in between breaths; don't try to inhale the water. Toss the cup toward a trash can or the side of the road without hitting another runner—this is a learned skill that requires some practice.

Refueling

Taking an energy gel while on the run is also a bit of a practiced art. Here are a few salient points:

- Squeeze as much into your mouth as possible. You may need to employ the "end of a toothpaste tube" trick and fold it up from the bottom to get every drop.
- Try not to get the sticky gel on your hands; it causes quite a mess.
- If possible, take a gel before nearing a water station, toss the empty packet in the trash and grab a water to help wash it down. If you're planning to walk at aid stations, that'd be a great time.

Since we're talking about a 10K, you may be fine taking an energy gel at the start and foregoing one on the course or use one around mile 4 to keep your energy up for the final 2.2 miles. I recommend you test this out in training to find what works best for you to keep your glycogen supply high and readily available.

Photographers & Finish Line

Brett's rule: Always run by a race photographer no matter how tired or sore you may feel. Unless you're actually injured, that photo will last a lot longer than your temporary discomfort! Because it's your first race, there's a good chance you'll keep it forever. The same thing holds true for the finish; summon every drop of your remaining willpower to finish strong with your head up high and a smile on your face.

After the finish line, make sure to keep moving while you grab some food and drink: a sports recovery drink with a 4:1 ratio of carbs to protein, a banana or a bagel with some peanut butter. By staying in motion as you cool down, you lessen the chances of cramping up. Once you've taken some nutrition, find a spot where you can perform some stretches and attempt to work some of the fatigue out of your legs, hips and glutes before enjoying the rest of the finish line expo and cheering on the other finishers.

Once you head home or back to your hotel, take a relaxing warm shower followed by a little quality time with a foam roller to loosen up your muscles and restore blood flow to limit soreness and kick-start recovery. A healthy meal 1–2 hours after your run is a great idea to replenish your glycogen stores as well as feed your muscles with protein and nutrients. I'll usually end a good race day with some celebratory frozen yogurt with my family, but that's up to you!

What's Next?

Congratulations on your race! Whether it was your first or fastest event, I sincerely hope you had a blast and reached your goal! The next move is entirely up to you, whether you want to move up from the Prep to the Level 1 Program and work on speed and power or continue using the program you're on with more intensity in order to improve your time—it's all within your grasp.

Remember, you can use these programs to successfully train for distances from 5K to 50K, so you can jump right back into the program with the exercises and drills you learned over the last seven weeks to propel you to racing new and challenging distances. The Level 1 and Level 2 programs are also an extremely effective way to get in killer shape as well as maintain your fitness and physique.

Whatever you choose, you can use these programs as a resource for developing your own program and hopefully building a long-term, healthy relationship with running that will pay dividends for the rest of your life. Share your passion for running with friends, family and loved ones. Who knows? You may become a coach and trainer yourself.

Thank you for allowing me to share my fitness journey with you. I sincerely hope you enjoyed reading it as much as I did living it and getting to write about it. If you have any questions, or suggestions, please feel free to contact me at www.7weekstofitness.com.

Progress Log

Use this log to track your progress throughout the program. Just photocopy as many copies of this page as you may need. For a downloadable version of this chart, visit www.7weekstofitness.com and click on the 7 Weeks to a 10K program. If you have a smartphone, you can download the mobile app from there as well.

Level_____	**Week**_____	start date_____
DAY	**DONE**	**EXERCISE NOTES (times, reps, exertion level, etc.)**
Mon	☐	
Tue	☐	
Wed	☐	
Thu	☐	
Fri	☐	
Sat	☐	
Sun	☐	

Photo Credits

Index